P9-EIF-277

"This book is like the act of riding a bike itself: easy, efficient, and fun. Essential reading for anyone contemplating cycling in a city — and for anyone already doing it."
— David Miller, Toronto mayor 2003–2010 and avid environmentalist

"*The Urban Cycling Survival Guide* is a comprehensive yet easy-to-read book that will enlighten you about all things urban cycling. Yvonne Bambrick is the perfect guide for any beginner cyclist."
— Mia Kohout, CEO and editor-in-chief of *Momentum Mag*

"Packed with useful tips and tricks, particularly for those new to urban cycling."
— Mia Birk, author of *Joyride: Pedaling Toward a Healthier Planet*

"From wearing a skirt or dress shoes to picking a bike to riding safely in traffic, *The Urban Cycling Survival Guide* breaks the basics of cycling down into manageable and understandable chunks helpful to novices and experienced cyclists. This is cycling for the every-person."
— Gabe Klein, former commissioner of Chicago and Washington, D.C., Department of Transportation and member of the NACTO Strategic Advisory Board

the URBAN CYCLING SURVIVAL Guide

NEED -TO- KNOW SKILLS & STRATEGIES for BIKING in the CITY

YVONNE BAMBRICK

Illustrated By MARC NGUI

ECW

Published by ECW Press
2120 Queen Street East, Suite 200, Toronto, Ontario, Canada M4E 1E2
416-694-3348 / info@ecwpress.com

Library and Archives Canada Cataloguing in Publication

Bambrick, Yvonne, author
      The urban cycling survival guide : need-to-know skills and strategies for biking in the city / Yvonne Bambrick; illustrations by Marc Ngui.

Issued in print and electronic formats.
ISBN 978-1-77041-218-7 (pbk)—ISBN 978-1-77090-709-6 (PDF)—ISBN 978-1-77090-710-2 (ePub)

      1. Cycling—Handbooks, manuals, etc. 2. City traffic—Handbooks, manuals, etc. I. Ngui, Marc, 1972–, illustrator II. Title.

GV1043.7.B34 2015   796.609173'2   C2014-907623-1
                                             C2014-907624-X

Editor for the press: Jennifer Knoch
Cover illustration and design: Marc Ngui
Interior photographs: Yvonne Bambrick
Author photo: © Javier Lovera

Printed and bound in Canada by Webcom   5   4   3   2   1

We acknowledge the financial support of the Government of Canada through the Canada Book Fund for our publishing activities, and the contribution of the Government of Ontario through the Ontario Book Publishing Tax Credit and the Ontario Media Development Corporation.

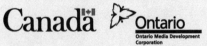

To my father, Timothy,
for taking me along on the ride,
and my mother, Barbara,
for nurturing my independent spirit.

Contents

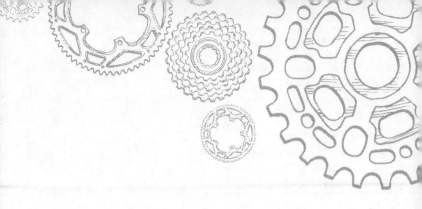

Introduction: Why Ride?

Bikes. Are. Everywhere. It doesn't take a study or statistic to prove that bicycle ridership is way up across North America — the sheer number of bicycles on the streets of your city, and even in upscale clothing store windows, is proof enough that the bike boom is upon us. Not since the 1890s have bikes been this cool. The timeless bicycle, once known as the mechanical or iron horse, is one of humanity's oldest manufactured self-propelled personal transportation vehicles, and one that's had a profound impact on our history. From its vital role in the emancipation of women and dramatic changes to their acceptable everyday clothing (hello, bloomers!) to the paving of our city streets, the first flight, and the widely accessible transportation of people and goods over ever-greater distances, the bicycle is nothing short of a two-wheeled wonder. Its classic design hasn't even changed much since 1885, when the safety bicycle, with two same-sized wheels, a drive chain, and inflated tires, was invented.

While most of our North American cities are in varying stages of adaptation to the bicycle (and yes, we're far from the bicycle nirvana of many European cities), millions of North Americans are choosing a bicycle for daily transportation. Gone are the days when bikes were seen as the last-resort transport of the poor or the domain of men in tight shorts and brightly coloured jerseys, a.k.a. MAMILs (middle-aged men in Lycra). Far more women and men of all ages, backgrounds, and occupations are now riding — and they're wearing whatever they like to do so. Bicycles are increasingly being seen, understood, and praised as the gloriously efficient, fun, fast, elegant, and accessible vehicles that they are — a classic solution to so many of the issues that seem to plague our cities. "When you ride your bike, it isn't just transportation, it is the key to designing the sustainable cities of the future," says Lloyd Alter, managing editor of TreeHugger.com.

With this growth in ridership, city governments across North America are also increasingly investing in expanded and updated bike infrastructure and programs, and they are recognizing bicycles as an important form of sustainable urban transportation that can help ease the burden of traffic congestion. While we might be on our way, we're not there yet: Interestingly, the most bike-friendly large city in North America, Portland, has the same bicycle ridership (6 per cent), as the least bike-friendly city in Germany, Stuttgart.

But as John Pucher and Ralph Buehler point out in their book *City Cycling*, with the right policies in place, levels of cycling can be dramatically increased: "Cities of all sizes with very different land use patterns, histories, and cultures have succeeded in increasing cycling and making it safer."

Unlike that found in the more-established cycling cities, North American transportation cycling culture is still growing and maturing; every year we have more riders with varying levels of skill. With a relatively young bike culture, limited bike-specific infrastructure (bike lanes, etc.), a gap in bike education, and a wider variety of riding conditions to adapt to, some cycling norms are still in development. New riders pick up cycling habits from watching others and through their own experiences. Although honing skills through observation and experience is important, it's crucial to start from a solid foundation of knowledge.

And that's where this book comes in. As a full-time cycling advocate, I noticed adults getting back on their bikes with only a partial understanding of how to be part of traffic on two wheels instead of four, or no understanding at all if they'd never gotten a driver's licence. The physical act of riding a bicycle — the balance and muscle movements needed to propel the vehicle forward — does come back quite easily. The part where you ride that bike out into the often fast-paced and shared vehicular roadways of your city is not quite so simple.

Although my first taste of independence was on my bicycle, like many, I felt the next level of freedom behind the wheel of the family car. I've been a licenced driver for over 20 years, and I actually quite like driving and can appreciate motor vehicles as the tools they are. I'm certain that being a cyclist first made me a better driver, and that being an occasional driver makes me a better cyclist, because it allows me to understand the roadway from both perspectives. I sold my Toyota Corolla in 2000 and used the money to pay for part of my post-graduate studies. Though I hadn't ridden much since my commute to and from high school, it didn't take me long to get back into the rhythm of the ride and realize what I'd been missing. The idea of buying a car hasn't crossed my mind since, and I've built my life in such a way that it shouldn't ever have to.

Getting back in the saddle allowed me to step back and see driving and car ownership from a whole new perspective. I realized that owning and habitually overusing a car for short trips actually made me and billions of others far more dependent on all the systems required to make, buy, park, insure, repair, and fuel a car, rather than providing the independence I'd originally connected to car ownership. Cars, while useful and essential to some, are also a factor in so many of our societal ills — obesity, stress, diseases related to a sedentary lifestyle, worsening air quality, urban sprawl, and divided communities to name but a few. Cars might be symbols of independence and freedom in advertising and rock anthems, but I've come to fully appreciate that bicycles actually provide it, and so much more.

I haven't written this book to convince you to become a full-time cyclist or give up driving. You are the only person who can make decisions about your daily transportation choices. My goal is to give you the information you need to be a confident rider whenever you choose: on weekends, once or twice a week, rain or shine — totally up to you.

But in case your conviction is wobbling like your bike on the first ride back, here are a few reminders of why it's worth braving those often daunting city streets on two wheels.

Convenience If you're used to a car, that might feel like the most convenient way to get around — you get in, turn on some tunes, and off you go. But how convenient is it to waste time in traffic or looking for parking?

A short trip by bike is almost always faster than one by car in an urban context, especially during rush hour. When you're in a hurry to get somewhere, there's nothing quite as satisfying, or motivating frankly, than effortlessly whipping past a long line of cars stuck in traffic. By the time they get through that last light, you've made it three blocks closer to your destination. Any busy person who is pressed for time can immediately see and feel the benefits of using a bicycle for getting around the city. Reduced and predictable travel time alone makes the bicycle a worthwhile, and minimal, investment. And if you can fit in a bit of easy cardio on your way to and from work, school, or errands, you've basically bought yourself more time for something else.

Autonomy Bikes are empowering, allowing you to get where you want to go on your own terms. You set your own pace and schedule, choose the door-to-door route you prefer, and kiss the malicious whims of transit delays and traffic jams goodbye. Also, don't underestimate the sense of accomplishment that comes from getting places on your own. Theatre-maker and songwriter Evalyn Parry says, "One of my cycling heroines is Frances Willard, the late 19th century women's suffrage leader of Evanston, Illinois, who put it so well in her 1895 book about cycling: 'She who succeeds in gaining mastery of the bicycle gains mastery of life.' Riding is so much about the pleasure of powering my own journey, moving at my own pace under my own steam."

A Healthier Body and Mind Cycling is a low-impact activity and is thus accessible to many people. Sure, you can put on sports clothes and go for a hard, fast ride to really get your heart pumping, but more often than not, riding a bike is a pretty easy form of exercise that you don't really notice you're doing — until you get to a hill, of course.

According to an Organisation for Economic Cooperation and Development (OECD) study on cycling health and safety, "Cycling significantly improves health and, as a form of moderate exercise, can greatly reduce clinical health risks linked to cardiovascular disease, Type-2 diabetes, certain forms of cancer, osteoporosis, and depression. . . . Not only does cycling reduce disease-related deaths, but it also contributes to substantially better health."

And if you're afraid the risks of urban cycling overshadow the benefits, the same study can help you rest easy: "On balance, the positive health impacts of cycling far outweigh the negative health impacts . . . including crash-related injuries and air pollution."

But it's not just about a healthy heart or legs of steel, says the OECD: "As well as improving physical health, cycling has a positive effect on emotional health — improving levels of well-being, self-confidence, and tolerance to stress while reducing tiredness, difficulties with sleep, and a range of medical symptoms."

Or take it from *Momentum Mag*'s CEO and editor-in-chief, Mia Kohout: "Riding a bike is my time of greatest reflection, creativity, and revelation. It is also a time when I get to slow down, breathe fresh air, and take in the sights, sounds, and smells of my city. Sometimes I don't feel like riding, so I don't, but I have never regretted it when I do."

We spend so much of our busy day sitting idly that it makes sense to mix exercise with something practical rather than trying to find time to get to the gym. As my good friend, local restaurant owner, and long-time cycling advocate Shamez Amlani is fond of saying, "Why drive to the gym, when you can ride to the restaurant?"

Money in Your Pocket Other than the initial investment in a bicycle and necessary accessories, usually somewhere between $200 and $2,500 depending on your means and needs, riding a bike for transportation is the cheapest way to go besides walking. A bike costs nearly nothing to ride, park, or fuel. You can do most basic maintenance yourself, and parts and repairs are

quite inexpensive. Say goodbye to your gym membership and slash your spending on public transit and taxis or gas, parking, and car repairs. If you go completely
car free, an increasingly popular choice in dense urban centres, you're also off the hook for monthly car
payments, maintenance, and insurance. According to
the U.S. Bureau of Transportation Statistics, the annual operating cost of a bike is from $308 to $821 (if you
include added food [i.e., fuel] costs due to increased
exercise) compared to the $8,220 to $11,000 it takes to
run a car.

Practical, Efficient Mobility The majority of trips we
take and errands we run in a day are under 5 kilometres (3 miles) from our home and perfectly suited to
travel by bike. In addition to its hyper-efficiency at con-
verting human energy into mobility, one of the greatest efficiencies of the bicycle is that it manages to fit
into and make use of tight spaces. Bikes can go places
cars can't — they are nimble, versatile, fast, slow, sturdy, and light. They're also just plain practical and can
allow you to experience your urban environment in a
whole new way.

(Re)Discovering Your City Whether you're new to your
city or have lived there your whole life, it can sur-
prise you when you see and feel it from two wheels.

Consultant Ken Greenberg writes, "For me, especially from the raised vantage point of a bicycle seat, the feeling is reminiscent of snorkelling. Like an exotic seascape seen from a fresh perspective, the city reveals itself in new ways. Self-propelled motion at relatively low speeds offers us more than exercise and a chance to commune with our neighbours. It restores a geographic intuition that was weakened by the car — a feel for the real distances between things, a sense of the connections between the parts of the city. It gives us back the ability to move through barriers between neighbourhoods and city districts, heedless of traffic volume or the many limits restricting where a car can go and when it can go there."

You also might end up spending more time in local businesses. Money spent on cars and fuel is mostly leaving your community, whereas cyclists and pedestrians put more money into local businesses. According to two studies done in Toronto (2009) and Portland (2012), customers arriving on bike or foot visit more often and spend more money cumulatively than car drivers.

Eco Warrior Cred We all know that bicycles have way less of an impact on our environment than cars — they cause no noise or air pollution, need no toxic batteries, and require fewer non-renewables to build, run, and maintain. Bicycles are far less implicated in the global oil industry and cause fewer resource extraction and waste concerns. This certainly makes me feel better as I make my way around my city, and never more so than on smog days when I know I'm not to blame for the bad air quality. In short, bicycles are the ultimate sustainable transportation vehicles.

Fun And if you weren't already convinced, let me just add that riding a bicycle is exhilarating. Who doesn't want to have fun on the way to work? Many people call their ride to and from work the best part of their day. Rather than adding to end-of-day fatigue, riding provides an energy boost after a long day.

So using a bike for transportation is cheap, efficient, practical, fun, convenient, and even healthy. Despite all those positives, riding in a fast-paced urban environment can still be intimidating. But remember, you don't need to jump in at full speed. Start on quiet side streets or on bike-specific paths, then work up to bike lanes and faster moving city roadways as your confidence grows. All city streets can become accessible to you by bike once you understand how to safely navigate them.

Each chapter addresses various aspects of urban cycling, from picking the right bike for your needs and learning the rules of the road to how to read other road users and navigate common obstacles. This is need-to-know stuff that might otherwise take you a long time to learn, often the hard way, through on-street practice and observation. While some of these details may already seem like common knowledge to you, they may be news to others. My goals are to give you a head start, or in some cases a reboot, in what will remain a daily learning experience and help you to better anticipate and appreciate the ups and downs of life on two wheels.

1

Gearing Up

Other than confidence and a good sense of how to behave as part of traffic, the only thing you need to get started cycling is a bicycle. You can begin by borrowing a bike or using a bike-share program if your city has one, but most people will soon want a ride of their own. It can be a bit overwhelming deciding which bicycle to pick, so in this chapter I'll be your guide to the bike styles and basic equipment you'll need to get you road-ready.

When I started riding regularly again in my early 20s, I went with an inexpensive used bike that a friend offered to me. It needed a repair, so with that (and a new lock) as the only expenses, I was off! I've since had about a half-dozen second-hand bikes that served their purpose but were nothing special. Each one was fairly generic looking and eventually either stolen or ridden beyond repair. In 2008, in part because of my new role as Toronto's cycling advocacy spokesperson, I got serious about the type of bike I was riding and picked up a life-changing (I'm not kidding) Dutch-style upright city bike. I currently have two bicycles — the Dutch bike, which serves as a workhorse for carrying groceries and any number of things, and a road-style city bike for longer distance or uphill rides when a lighter, faster bike makes it a bit easier going.

There are several basic bike styles and many models to choose from, but the easiest way to start is talking with friends who ride and shopping around online. Next, find the nearest bike shops and visit them to see, feel, and try out what they've got in stock. Researching through friends and online means that you can be better prepared when you get there and know what you want to try out. Even if your budget only allows you to pick up a bike from a large chain retailer, visiting independent bike shops can give you a better sense of the bike landscape, and they are a good place to ask "bikey" questions. If you continue to ride regularly, chances are you'll eventually want to upgrade your wheels, and independent bike shops are the place to do so. Bike shops can be fantastic community hubs and a great source of all kinds of bike-related information. It's not uncommon to build a strong connection to a particular bike shop that you find welcoming.

Eric Kamphof of Toronto's Curbside Cycle says, "My job is to link new city cyclists with that object that makes them a cyclist: their bike. So much has to do with the bike. A city has a certain pace, a beat, and a city bike rides in tune with that beat, keeping you upright, aware, and a beautiful part of the landscape. So much of the success of Paris's Velib bike share program, or New York's Citi bike has to do with the bike itself. Take one ride and the world just opens up. You don't just feel safe, you feel free. That's what a city bike does, it empowers you, it demythologizes all the fears put upon city cycling and reveals the uncomplicated joyfulness that it is."

You don't need to be a "cyclist" to ride a bike. The term is just a convenient way to refer to someone using a bicycle.

But how do you find a good, honest bike shop? Zack Stender, co-owner of San Francisco's Huckleberry Bicycles, advises asking around: "A shop with a knowledgeable staff and a strong selection of bikes in the type you are looking for will do wonders for your shopping experience. Also, not all bike shop service departments are equal, so you would be well advised to patronize a shop with a reputable mechanic staff. Online reviews can be helpful but talking to other folks who ride is best. Ask other cyclists which shops they prefer, and when you visit these locations follow your gut."

Bike shops are primarily in the business of selling and repairing bikes, and they can get ridiculously busy from spring through fall, in particular in cities with harder winters. So with that in mind, unless you have an urgent repair, try to time your visit based on your needs and their schedule. If you're not sure what seasons or days are more busy or less busy, ask the staff. You can be pretty sure that there will be less people stopping in on a rainy day (unless, of course, you live in a very rainy city), and equally certain that the first nice spring weekend after a cold winter will be a gong-show that is best avoided. Fall is usually a great time of year to buy a bike, as many are on sale near the end of the season — the new year brings the latest models. Shops may have less selection, but they'll be less busy.

Keep an eye open for bicycle trade shows — they're a great chance to meet the local retailers, ask questions, see what models are going to be available for the new year, and test out different styles of bicycles all in one place. You'll be able to place an order if you find a bike you like.

Before you actually take the plunge and pick up your ride, there are several things to consider.

Budget What do you currently spend monthly for transportation? How often do you think you'll ride your bike instead of taking public transit? If you're going to be driving less and riding more, how much will you save on gas, parking, tickets, and time if you ride two, three, or five days a week in weather you're comfortable riding in? Remember, you get what you pay for. A good bike is worth the investment. Assuming you do everything you can to keep your bike safe from theft, you'll probably have it for several years — let's say five years for this budgeting exercise. Add up the money you estimate you'll save every year by riding, multiply it by five, and then divide it in half. That's more than enough to pay for a great bike that suits your needs. You may not have this money at the ready now, but this exercise is meant to put what seems like an expensive purchase into perspective. Don't forget to allocate a bit of money for necessary accessories like a lock. (Read more about accessories later in this chapter.)

Distance of Travel Something for long weekend rides or just for short daily errands? If you're commuting, how many kilometres (or miles) will you log daily? Travelling longer distances often means you'll want a lighter bike, but you'll also have to factor in terrain and speed:

◇ What's the terrain like where you'll be riding? Paved city streets or the nearby park trail? Mostly flat, hilly, or a bit of both? Are there many potholes in your city or are the roads well maintained?

◇ Are you planning to try to keep up with car traffic, move swiftly but carefully, or take a slow and steady approach? It should be noted that safely keeping up with regular fast-moving car traffic takes time and practice. Doing so with little on-street cycling experience can be bad news.

Parking and Storage Where will you be storing and parking your bike, overnight in particular, at home and at your main destinations? Do you have access to a garage at home or secure indoor bike parking at your office? Do you live in an apartment and plan to bring your bike inside? Is there an elevator available and does your building allow bikes inside and on the elevator? Will you be leaving your bike locked up outside? If you need to carry your ride up a flight of stairs, for example, a light bike will be a priority. Trust me when I say that doing this twice daily, or more, in particular if you have a load on your bike, will take a toll on your body. If you are bringing your bike indoors and into an elevator, always remember to be conscientious of others by making space for them and keeping dirty tires away from people's clothing and from walls.

MEET YOUR MATCH: FINDING THE BIKE FOR YOU

The bicycles that fill our cities are as diverse and colourful as the people riding them. There are, however, some basic styles to choose from, and this list should help you discover what type of bike might work best for you.

Road Bike Designed with speed and longer distance road travel in mind, these bikes usually have a sleek, light frame; smooth, thin tires; and position the rider so that the upper body is out front and down to reduce

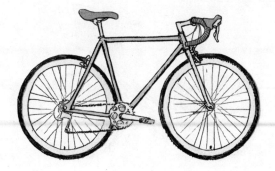

wind resistance. This position requires you to hold your head up and back so that you can see properly, and it can be uncomfortable for your neck and lower back. Gearing provides many speed options, allowing you to adjust to terrain and navigate steep inclines. Though road bikes are the best choice for speed, high speeds in a race position can be unsafe in busy mixed traffic. You generally want to have your head up so that you can see everything coming your way. Some people are also less comfortable with the skinny tires. That said, road bikes are a preference for confident riders for whom speed and the ability to easily cover longer distances are of highest importance.

City or Upright Bike The European-style (or Dutch-, English-, or Italian-style) city bike is designed as a practical everyday bike for commuting and year-round use. These bikes often have a step-through frame (with a

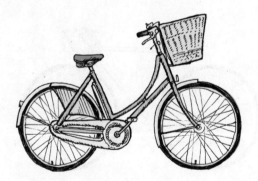

top tube that dips down), which makes getting on and off easier, and a rear rack, skirt guard, chain guard, built-in lights, a rear wheel lock, and a comfortable tall handlebar position. The rider sits in a sturdy upright position, allowing good visibility and sightlines. Some are single speed for extra simplicity on flatter terrain, while others have gears, often internal, which help with small hills. Higher-end city bikes also often have internal hub brakes, which can perform better when the weather is nasty.

Mountain Bike With a thicker frame and wheels, knobbly tires, and a more upright riding position, this is a steed made for off-road riding on uneven terrain, whether it's forest trails or urban roads that ride like rumble strips. This style is less efficient for urban commuting — it may handle rough roads a bit better, but the tires can slow you down on longer commutes.

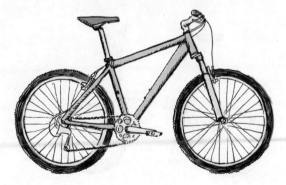

Hybrid This popular choice for city riding has a thicker, more robust frame and wheels than a road bike, providing riders with a less hunched-over position, though not quite as upright as a city bike. The tires have grip but are faster than those of a mountain bike.

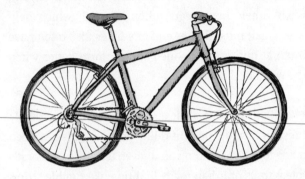

Folding Bike These nifty transformers are a fantastic option if you want to easily bring your bike indoors or onto public transit. Some are easier than others to

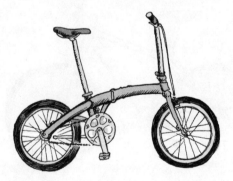

collapse and reset, but smaller wheels don't have too much impact on speed for regular rides across the city. There are various styles, features, and levels of functionality.

Cruiser Primarily used for recreation, these bikes are often more stylish. With extra-thick tires and a wide, relaxed handlebar position, choose this model for relaxed weekend rides rather than daily commutes.

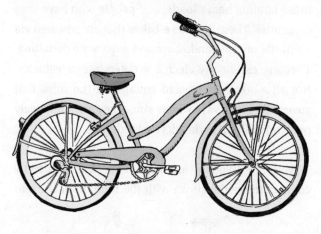

Electric Assist Bike (or Pedelec) These bicycles have an integrated battery that provides extra power to the rider when they pedal, and they come in various models and styles. However, many regular bicycles can be fitted with an electric battery boost that can assist the rider in propelling the bicycle. This can be particularly

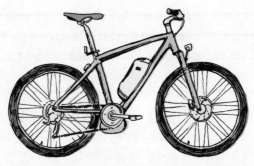

helpful for older riders, people with mobility issues, those hauling heavy loads, and people who have long commutes. There are also **e-bikes** that are powered via a throttle on the handlebars and require no pedalling. They are essentially electric scooters/motor vehicles. Not all e-bikes are created equal, and the rules that govern their use vary widely since they are a relatively new (re)addition to the bicycle landscape.

Fixed-Gear Bike Not for beginners, "fixies" directly connect the pedal stroke with the rotation of the rear

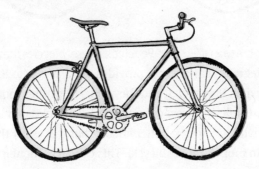

wheel via a drive chain. Unlike regular bicycles, which allow a rider to stop pedalling at will thanks to a free-wheel system, fixed-gear bikes require resistance on the pedals to slow or stop the bike once in motion. Limited parts do mean less maintenance, and some appreciate the increased connection to the movement of the wheels.

STEEL VS. ALUMINUM

The material used for a bike frame is important too. Aluminum is lighter and more stiff than steel. But while steel is heavier, it's also better able to absorb shocks from uneven and bumpy city streets. The importance of shock absorption should not be underestimated, and the durability of steel likely means your bike will last longer.

There are various other styles of bicycles, and some are more suited to older riders, those with mobility issues, and those who ride with children. (See Chapter 5 for more information.)

Bike Fit

A well-fitted bicycle can make a huge difference, so even if you choose to buy your first bike from a large retailer instead of a bike shop, be sure to ask for help getting the best fit. There are several factors that affect bike fit.

Frame Size Bike frames come in various sizes, so you want to be sure to get the one that best suits your body. When you straddle the bike frame, not sitting on the seat but with it behind you and your feet on the ground, the top tube should be about 2.5 centimetres (1 inch) away from your crotch. Ideally, you should be able to stand comfortably without the frame coming into contact with your body. This measurement only matters if you're buying a bike with a top tube, of course. There are also step-through frames, which don't have a tube across the top and are easier to get on and off. Step-throughs usually come in a couple of different sizes suited to a range of heights.

Handlebar Height and Placement As part of getting your bicycle fitted correctly, check the distance you have to reach when seated. Your arms should be slightly bent at the elbows and not overextended. Seats can be moved a few centimetres (or a couple of inches) back or forward if you need smaller adjustments. You also don't want to put too much weight on your hands. Are your wrists comfortable? Although handlebar styles are generally dictated by the style of bicycle, you can swap them out for something more comfortable. When the handlebars are higher than the seat, such as on Dutch- and some commuter-style bikes, you generally have a more comfortable and relaxed ride. A seat that's at the same height as, or slightly higher than, the handlebars puts you in more of a racing position. This is more aerodynamic, but it can also lead to neck strain. The more upright your upper body is when riding in the city the better, for your back, visibility, sightlines, and overall comfort, including your comfort in the saddle.

Seat Style and Height Your seat can be moved in three different ways. You can move it up or down so that you're sitting at the right height — ideally you want your knee to be slightly bent when you've reached the bottom of the pedal stroke while seated. A super straight leg, or overextended knee, means your seat is too high; a deep bend in your knee means it's too low.

Seats can be shifted forward and back to move you a bit closer to or further from the handlebars.

Finally, the seat can tilt up and down. Most of your weight should rest on your sit bones. Women's sit bones are generally further apart than men's, which means that wider seats are often better suited to women. A poor saddle fit isn't only uncomfortable: According to recent research findings out of Yale, too much pressure on a women's perineum can have negative impacts on genital sensation over time — and that's a sure way to make riding less sexy. Since similar findings exist for the impact of such seat pressure on men, we all need to keep it in mind.

Your bike will come with a standard seat/saddle, but there are other options available that may suit you better. For example, I was struggling with a kink in my neck for a while. It wasn't until I spent a week riding around in a less bumpy city and the kink went away that I realized I needed a bike seat that could help absorb the shock of our bumpy roads. Replacing the seats on both of my bikes with new spring-loaded hard leather saddles has made riding so much more enjoyable! A good saddle is even more important if you're doing long rides quite regularly. Riding should never be a pain in the butt.

Sealing the Deal: Advice Before Buying

When you're deciding on what bike to buy, take time to test ride different styles to see what feels the best for you. Bike shops will ask you to leave collateral — generally your credit card or some form of ID. Get the seat height adjusted and then go for a ride around the block a few times. If you're able to take it for a longer ride, even 10 minutes, you'll get a really good feel for how you settle into the bike. A longer ride is definitely recommended once you've narrowed down the bikes you're considering. Bring a friend if you're nervous.

On your test ride be sure to

◊ try the gears to see how they work and feel,

◊ test the brakes carefully,

◊ make a few turns in both directions,

◊ practise getting on and off the bike.

You should also take note of how your body feels when you're riding — is your back straight, are the handlebars too close or far, is the seat comfortable and at the right height?

Once you've settled on a bike, be sure to ask for details about the warranty at the shop you're buying it from. The shop may include free tune-ups for a year or more as a purchase incentive and welcome you back after a week or two of riding your new bike so that any adjustments can be made — tightening up loose bits, adjusting the height of your handlebars, or shifting your seat for greater comfort.

Used Bikes

Used bikes can be a great option if you have limited funds, want to reduce your environmental footprint, or are just flirting with urban cycling. As with new bikes, you want to check the bike fit. Do your research at local bike shops about the shape, style, and frame size that is best suited to your body and riding goals before heading out to look for a second-hand bike.

When you do find a bike that might be right for you, you'll want to give it a good once-over. Don't buy it if

◊ there are bends in the dropouts (the point where the wheels are attached to the frame);

◊ the seat post has become fused in place and can't move up or down;

◊ there are any big dents or cracks in the frame;

◊ any of the welds where the various parts of the bike are joined are cracked or unstable;

◊ the bottom bracket (where the pedal arms meet at the frame) is rattling or loose.

If the frame and key components are in good shape, you can repair or replace wheels that are out of true (bent), brakes or tires that are worn down, or a seat that is cracked. If you're able, it's always helpful to bring along a friend, bike savvy or not, when shopping for a bike, new or used.

Now this probably isn't news to you, but bike theft is one of the biggest problems faced by bike owners. This means that not only do you need to take care when locking up your bike, you need to be extra careful about buying a used or second-hand bike because there's a possibility that it's stolen property.

So where does that leave you? Check out

◊   bike shops: some sell second-hand bikes, and they are usually careful about who they get them from;

◊   police department auctions, where items recovered by police are sold to the public;

◊   garage sales;

◊   DIY bike collectives that sell bikes or can help you make your own bike with parts and offer guidance;

◊   online sites like Craigslist, but be careful about buying this way and trust your instincts about the seller (online or in person) — if the deal seems too good to be true or the seller seems kind of dodgy, steer clear.

Add-ons

Before you hit the road, there are at least three additional purchases that you should make at the same time as you buy your bike.

A **good lock** is almost more important than the bike you decide on. I use two different locks at once and recommend you do the same. The prices on locks vary widely, and they can go from cheap at $15 to solid and much more dependable at around $180. See the Bike Theft section in Chapter 3 for more details on how to keep your bike safe.

Lights are required for riding at night and just make sense. (For more on light laws, see pages 92–93.)

A **bell** is needed any time you ride to help communicate with others around you. Some cities, like Edmonton, New York, and Washington, DC, require a bell or a horn by law, while others strongly recommend getting them for your bike as a safety precaution. In general, a bell is a tool that every urban rider should have on their bike; they aren't particularly expensive, and they're extremely handy. Even with a bell in place, don't be afraid to speak up to alert people of your presence or communicate your intentions to other road users.

Some bikes, like my city bike, come with lights and a bell attached and a rear wheel lock, but generally you are required to purchase these things separately.

A **helmet** is required by law in some parts of North America. Cities like Vancouver and Seattle mandate helmets by law. Other cities use age restrictions: Toronto and Calgary require only cyclists under the age of 18 to wear a helmet, whereas New York City mandates helmets for cyclists 13 years old and younger.

Many people prefer to ride with a helmet even with no law in place; however, helmet use is one of the most contentious elements of bike riding. If you fall and hit your head, that brain bucket might help you out. In a 2012 research paper summary, the *Canadian Medical Association Journal* suggests, "Not wearing a helmet while cycling was associated with an increased risk of dying as a result of sustaining a head injury." This means that of the cases studied, more people survived a head injury because they'd been wearing a helmet in the crash.

While helmets can, in some cases, help diminish the harm that may occur in a fall or collision, they do nothing to prevent those falls or collisions from occurring — cycling isn't inherently dangerous, but the conditions on our North American city streets often are. Some argue, based on studies such as one published in 2011 by the Society for Risk Analysis in Virginia, that wearing a helmet can cause a rider to take greater risks because of a greater sense of security. Another study, out of the University of Bath, concluded that drivers generally leave less space when passing a rider with a helmet because of the perceived protection provided to the rider by the helmet.

While helmets can and do reduce injuries in certain types of crashes and collisions, making them mandatory, as in Australia, has been shown to reduce cycling numbers. All cyclists are safer when more people are out riding, with or without helmets.

The use of a helmet while riding is a very personal matter, and unless clearly listed as a legal requirement where you ride, it's up to you to decide whether using one is what works best for you. Some people feel safer and more confident with a helmet on, while others feel the same without one.

If you're going to wear a helmet, make sure you get a good one, approved by the relevant safety organizations in the U.S. or Canada (listed in the sidebar). A good fit is also crucial: A loose or ill-fitting helmet will not work properly in a crash and will move around on your head more than necessary, likely resulting in extra-bad helmet hair. All bike helmets should sit flat on your head, as opposed to tilting backward or forward. The straps should be snugly secured to form a V — loose straps mean a loose helmet. Buckle the chinstrap securely so that only two fingers can fit between the strap and your chin. Helmets come in a wide variety of styles, shapes, and colours, so you should be able to find one that's your favourite colour or matches your bike.

It is generally recommended that you replace any helmet involved in a crash. If you've hit your head, the helmet will have absorbed some of the impact and may not be as effective in any future crashes. If in doubt, take it in to a local bike shop and ask for advice or contact the manufacturer. And, for these reasons, be extra careful about buying a helmet second-hand: If it shows any signs of impact, take a pass.

There are many other add-ons that can be purchased at bike shops that aren't strictly essential but can make your ride much more pleasant. Prices will

HELMET CERTIFICATION

U.S.

As of 1999, all bicycle helmets manufactured in, or imported to, the U.S. must meet federal safety standards set by the Consumer Product Safety Commission (CPSC). The CPSC website maintains a handy pamphlet detailing its standards for all sport helmets. Urban cyclists should look for any of the following CPSC approvals in any helmets they purchase:

» CPSC

» ASTM F1447

» Snell B-90/95

» Snell N-94†

Canada

According to the Ontario Ministry of Transportation website, and also applicable across Canada, helmets should have a sticker on the inside signalling certifying safety standards from the following organizations:

» Canadian Standard Association: CAN/ CSA D113.2-M89

» Snell Memorial Foundation: Snell b90, Snell B90s, or Snell n94

» American National Standard Institute: ANSI z90.4-1984

» American Society for Testing and Materials: ASTMF1447-94

» British Standards Institute: BS6863:1989

» Standards Association of Australia: AS2063.2-1990

vary, as always, based on quality and materials. Since different shops tend to carry different products, it's worth shopping around to find what you like best. Your bike will eventually become an extension of you. Over time you'll make adaptations and additions to personalize it to your needs and habits.

When used properly, **kickstands** ($10 to $35) hold your bike upright and allow you to let go of the bike without it falling over. This can be particularly handy when there is no wall or sturdy object to rest your bike against or when you're taking things out of your panniers (carry bags) or loading them. Some parking situations require the kickstand to be used so that your bike stays up. While most kickstands are a single arm mounted on one side of the bike, some are V shaped and come down on both sides of the bottom bracket, where the pedals are attached. This style is generally more sturdy but lifts the front wheel off the ground completely — not your best option if you have a front basket because the extra weight can make the front end flip sideways. Not all kickstands are created equal, so be sure to pick one up that is robust enough to properly support your bike.

Skirt or wheel guards are amazing and can keep any long apparel from getting caught up in the spokes or rear brakes. These come standard on Dutch-style city bikes but can be added to just about any bike. They fit over the rear wheel and usually cover both sides of

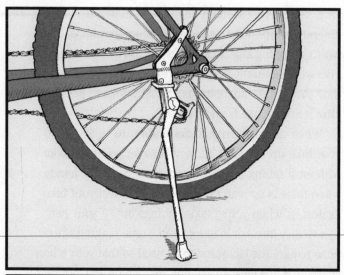

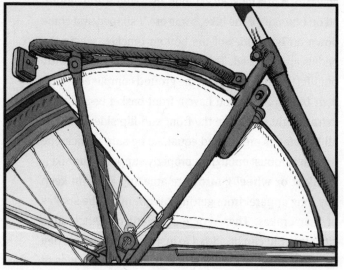

the top quarter of the wheel closest to where you are positioned on the bike seat. While you can purchase a wheel guard ($25 to $100), you can also make one yourself out of fabric, and there are DIY tutorials online to show you how.

Most bikes have an exposed chain that requires you to either roll up your right pant leg, tuck it into your sock, or use something to strap it down. **Chain guards** ($25 to $150) cover your chain instead. Some cover only the top and front portion of the chain, leaving the bottom exposed and your pants vulnerable, while others fully enclose the chain in a way that protects it from the elements, road salt, and grit and protects you from the chain. Not all bikes are built to accommodate a chain guard, but they're worth the small investment if yours can fit one.

I'd never ride a bike in the city without **mud guards or fenders** ($25 to $150). Mud guards are mounted on the top/rear side of both the front and rear wheels and keep grit, water, mud, and other things (like garbage sludge) off you — guaranteeing a cleaner, and happier, ride. Many bikes come standard with these attached, but otherwise you'll need to find the ones that are best suited to the bike you have in mind by asking at the local bike shop.

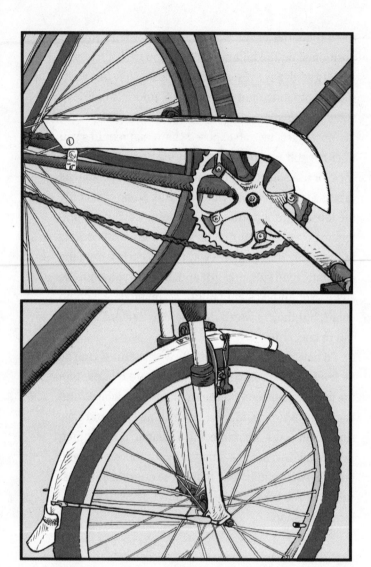

Adding Carrying Capacity

The best thing I ever did was attach a front basket and rear rack to my bicycle. Having a quick and easy spot to carry something while riding is super handy and is totally worth the small investment. And best of all, no more sweaty back! But there are tons of ways to turn your bike into a regular beast of burden, so read on to find an option that works best for you.

Front baskets come in many shapes, sizes, and materials and are not just for women. They can range in price from $15 to $80, and some of us do like to decorate ours with flowers, but this is certainly not a requirement.

Front baskets are a great place to stash small bags and purses — especially anything containing valuables, since you can keep them in your line of sight. A front basket can take some getting used to since it adds weight to your handlebars, but it doesn't take long to adjust. Front baskets are better suited to some bikes. A road bike, for example, works well with a rear rack onto which panniers can be attached.

More bikes than ever are available with a **rear rack** built in as part of the design, but it is still generally something that has to be purchased separately. Prices range from $15 to $140 based on materials, style, and function (weight capacity). When you consider just how useful it can be, even the most basic rack is a totally worthwhile addition.

Rear racks are designed primarily as the place onto which you can attach panniers and **rear baskets**. But, even if you never buy or use one of these attachable items, the rack itself can do a lot of work for you. For example, you can use a bungee cord, or two, to strap down your backpack so that the bike carries the weight instead of your back.

Panniers vary widely in price and are basically backpacks adapted to clip onto and hang from a rear, or sometimes front, bike rack. There are fixed and detachable panniers, and they come in a wide range of styles, materials, and prices. My preference is a waterproof pannier, for when you're caught in the rain and don't want to worry about the electronics or paperwork you've got along on your ride. Since starting to carry my laptop in both my removable and fixed panniers, I've added extra padding to the compartment where the laptop is stowed to help absorb the shocks from going over bumps and potholes and to reduce any impact on my electronics.

Most **detachable panniers** have a shoulder strap in addition to a simple handle. Some pannier clips are fiddlier than others, so be sure to physically test out the attaching and detaching action required before purchasing one.

Fixed panniers, such as the ones I have on my

upright city bike, usually come in pairs and have a joining strap that goes across and affixes to the top of the back rack. You might think these would get stolen and that you always want to take your panniers with you, but, surprisingly, I've never once had them stolen or even lost something that I've left inside them. That said, you probably don't want to leave anything of value in them unattended. Fixed and collapsible metal pannier baskets are also a great option as they can be neatly folded down and kept out of the way. The nice thing about fixed panniers is that they're always there when you need them — sort of like the trunk of a car.

Under seat bags ($10 to $35) are designed to fit right underneath your seat and usually strap onto the metal frame of the seat. Many people use these to store tire patch kits and basic bike tools (see Chapter 4 for more details on maintenance and tools). These are usually left in place on the bike.

When you carry anything on a bike, your main concern should be to keep any part of the load from dangling and getting stuck or tangled in your wheels, brakes, or spokes. So, plastic bags over handlebars . . . not a great idea. You also want to get whatever it is to wherever you're going in one piece. **Bungee cords** ($1–$15) are an essential, inexpensive, and versatile tool for strapping down things on any vehicle, but on a bike in particular. Do be careful while using a bungee — the cord is under pressure and can cause damage if the tension is released unexpectedly. My bikes always have one attached to the rear rack or sitting in the bottom of my pannier at the ready. Hardware shops, dollar stores, and even gas stations carry these. They come in different lengths and have several styles of hooks, and the quality also varies. However you load up your bike, and you'd be amazed at just how many different things you can carry on one, make sure it's as balanced as possible.

Wide ranging in style and priced from $1,200 to $5,000, **cargo bikes** are designed specifically to carry large loads of goods of any kind as well as other people, children in particular. In traditional cargo bikes, known as bakfiets (box bikes), the loads go in a basin that is part of an extended frame in front of the handlebars, but others (known as longtails or midtails) have an extended rear wheel base and rack section. There are also bakfiets that, although heavier, offer additional stability with two front wheels, and various other rear box styles have recently been introduced.

North Americans have far more options now that cargo bikes have come back into favour as a great alternative to the automobile — there are many styles to choose from based on your needs. Zack Stender, co-owner of San Francisco's Huckleberry Bicycles, has been watching the trend: "The culture is strong and only growing. These bikes, though they tend to lose a bit of their zippiness and weigh a bit more than a standard bike, pay off in loading capacity and make these a perfect option for those who like the ideas of self-sufficiency and human power. Who needs a car when you can carry 200 pounds [90 kilograms] of gear and kids on your beautiful bicycle?" And if hauling large loads seems daunting, for $800 to $1,500 you can also add electric assist to make getting started and going up inclines a bit easier.

Bike trailers are a fantastic option for adding a large temporary carrying capacity to your bike, particularly for hauling children (see Chapter 5), and can run from $150 to $1,000. Some bike trailers are 3 metres (10 feet) long and used for things like moving house! Others are more like a golf caddy and hook up onto your seat post. If you regularly need to carry a specific type of load, you can have a custom bike trailer made, or just shop around for the one that best suits your needs. Ready-made bike trailers can also be modified to fit the type of load you need to carry. Some local bike organizations now loan or rent them out, so you don't necessarily need to invest in your own if you only need one from time to time. Different trailers respond various ways to turns, and some are more stable when they're loaded. If you do borrow or rent a bike trailer, be sure to ask for training on how to use it properly.

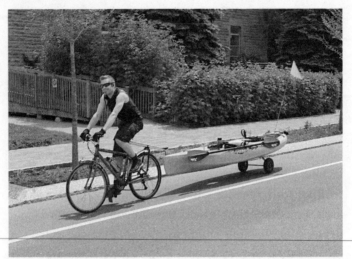

You can haul just about anything by bike!

What to Wear

A bike, and how you wear it, ride it, and use it, is a reflection of your personality, your taste, and you as an individual. If you've got a certain look, you can play it up while riding. I have a couple of male friends who rarely leave the house without a fedora — there's nothing quite as dapper as a man on a bike in a hat and jacket.

As it was in the late 1800s, women's bike fashion is still a popular topic in bicycle circles. "I ride my city bike (a Bobbin Birdie with a basket) to business meetings, galas, weddings, funerals, you name it," says April Economides, president of Green Octopus Consulting. "I love this mostly because it feels joyful and freeing — but I also like to show folks that yes, dressed-up women do ride bikes. When my grandpa died, I rode my bike to his funeral at his Greek Orthodox church in the requisite fancy all-black attire, and it was immensely healing to arrive and leave the service that way. In fact, it has been the most impactful part of my healing process to date."

Turning heads isn't just about vanity; other road users tend to notice a nicely put together outfit. Of course, nice outfits are harder to see at night, so don't forget your bike lights. Toronto's Deadly Nightshades Bike Crew even finds ways to make flashy fashionable: "We love the idea of visibility and bike safety being something that's fun and stylish, not something that feels like a chore. We like cutting up 3M tape to make reflective fringe, wearing crazy patterns, lots of bling and high heels. Staying safe and looking rad don't need to be mutually exclusive."

Sometimes wearing clothing and gear that is specifically designed for physical activity and/or cycling is more appropriate. Try layering key pieces of sportswear under or over your regular clothes, or just bring a change of clothes and pull a quick change when you get to your destination. Many people with longer cycling commutes find it far more comfortable to wear things like padded bike shorts, padded gloves, jerseys that wick away sweat, and wind-resistant jackets.

While I usually just wear what I'd wear if I was taking any other mode of transport, there are some bike specific things to consider with clothing choices:

◊ I tend to tie long skirts or dresses in one or two side-knots and also keep a large binder clip on my bike that comes in handy for holding certain skirt styles in place. Check out PennyInYour Pants.co.uk for another great riding trick for skirts.

◊ Non-padded bike shorts under a skirt can preserve your modesty and stop the skirt from being a distraction while you ride.

◊ Keep pant legs strapped tight to your legs with a Velcro or metal pant strap or rolled up to avoid chain grease. Reflective Velcro pant straps are handy for many things and can become an essential part of your bike kit.

◊ Low-rise jeans call for a long top so that your butt doesn't stick out when bending forward to ride.

◊ Your eyes are exposed to the wind, weather, and debris while riding. Wearing sunglasses during the day and clear glasses during inclement weather, or on longer rides at night, can help protect your eyes and maintain visibility.

◊ On longer rides, padded bike gloves protect your hands from calluses and help maintain good grip when your hands heat up and get sweaty. You can also use the back of your glove to wipe sweat from your face.

◊ Footwear is worth considering since your shoe is the direct link between you and your bicycle power. Keep in mind things like grip, slip, comfort, warmth, dryness, and overall safety. For example, flip-flops are not ideal footwear while riding; they might do for a short dash to the corner store but not for your daily commute. Shoelaces should be properly tied and can be tucked into your shoe or under the crossed laces.

◊ Whatever you can do to increase your visibility is a good thing. Lighter and brighter colours can help, and there are more sport clothing options than ever before that offer reflective elements. A reflective sash over your suit jacket can make all the difference and is easy to keep in your purse, pannier, or pocket. On cold nights I've often worn my safety vest over my stylish winter coat when en route. It gets stashed in my purse on arrival.

◊ Work clothes can be rolled up (the best strategy for keeping them wrinkle free) and carried along in a waterproof pannier for long and sweaty or rainy rides. Allowing five to ten minutes for a quick change will leave you fresh and ready for your workday.

In short, if you can wear it on your walk or drive to work, you can almost certainly wear it on your ride. Initially you may face some psychological barriers: fear of sweat, fear of looking unkempt, fear of being uncomfortable, fear of being smelly, soggy, etc. I've found that giving over to occasional, temporary, and usually minimal discomfort is inevitably rewarded by the benefits of arriving on time, with an endorphin boost and the knowledge that I am a self-sufficient person — independence and freedom trump rain in my face or sweat on my brow. But packing a change of clothes and keeping a stick of deodorant in your bag can give you peace of mind.

2

Navigating the Streetscape

City traffic is a fluid and unpredictable beast. The movement along our streets presents a series of choices we need to make regardless of our mode of transport, but we need to make even more choices from the seat of a bicycle. The more you ride, the better a decision-maker you'll become regarding what risks are acceptable while navigating through the daily urban obstacle course. Riding assertively, anticipating what's ahead, and selecting the right route are all keys to making cycling a fantastic way to get around the city.

Your vulnerability is real on a bicycle and shouldn't be underestimated. Be prepared to adapt to situations as they arise en route, and understand that riding a bike as part of traffic requires continuous adjustments to stay balanced and in control. As Robert Hurst writes in *The Cyclist's Manifesto*, "Bicycling demands coordination, fluidity of motion, and quickness of reflexes far beyond what is necessary for driving. . . . Bicycling requires a certain minimal sum of skill and spirit. If you're low on skill . . . you need to be strong in other ways to make up for it."

This chapter will give you a good sense of the types of things that you can expect to come across, tips on how to handle them, ways to better read and understand the roadway landscape, a sense of your responsibility in the mix, and how to avoid various hazards. Drawing from the regulations in 20 major cities in Canada and the U.S., I'll also share the most common laws for urban cyclists, but it's always good to look into the specific regulations in your city.

These rules and guidelines for urban cycling are a great foundation upon which you can add your own lived-and-learned experience. If you're new to everyday utilitarian/commuter cycling, consider taking a cycling skills development workshop. The more you ride, the more you'll learn about what type of rider you are, what types of situations you feel comfortable in, the types of streets you prefer, and those to avoid. Go at your own pace and try not to let minor setbacks, falls, or collisions stop you from riding. Every one of the riders you see out on the road has experienced something similar. As with most things in life, there are bumps, bruises, and scary bits along the way to becoming a confident and independent urban cyclist.

"Relax; forget what you thought about city riding," advises Noah Budnick, deputy director of Transportation Alternatives in New York City. "Think about your city and what you love about it. Ride. Re-experience your city and what makes it special to you — the bike will help you see what you love about it from a new perspective. Before anyone gets on a bike, they need to imagine themselves riding a bike."

If you come across a situation that makes you uncomfortable or unsure, you can always get off your bike and walk it along the sidewalk until you are past the issue.

Being safe on the roadway comes down to one thing: staying alert and aware at all times. If you love to daydream or get lost in your thoughts while moving from A to B, riding a bike for transportation may not be for you. I have a very close friend who came to this realization, and as much as I miss being able to ride places together, she made the decision that's safest for her. Weekend recreational riding on park paths or other off-road routes is still an excellent option if you can't stay über attentive, responsive, and focused on the road and everything happening around you during a typical commute.

Safe cycling is all about predicting what could happen in the roadway in front of you through constant and keen observation, scanning in all directions and then responding appropriately to whatever occurs along your ride. This vigilance can be broken down into four basic maxims:

1. **Scan** everything in your field of vision ahead of you on the road — move your eyes back and forth across the entire streetscape. You want to be looking at not just the road and cars in front of you on the road, but also at the parked cars, the movements of pedestrians, upcoming driveways, cars turning onto the street, blind spots behind larger parked or moving vehicles, etc.

2. **Anticipate** what types of things could happen as you move through the streetscape and roadway. For example, consider that pedestrian who is looking down at his phone, listening for cars but not looking for bikes, and whose body language suggests he might jaywalk at the next "gap in traffic" or the driver ahead of you that is slowing down mid-block near a driveway — she hasn't signalled a turn, but might turn anyway.

3. **Evade** any anticipated movements or unexpected interactions as safely and carefully as possible. If you've anticipated something, you should be able to shift lanes or your lane position, adjust your speed, and signal if necessary to avoid the issue. Unexpected interactions usually require a quick reaction, but they don't always allow time for you to signal your intentions. We'll get into signals and communication on page 55–57.

4. **Correct** your lane position and riding speed after you've manoeuvred the obstacle safely. Remember to also breathe and try to relax, but don't let your guard down. Keep scanning and always remain focused and aware of what's happening around you.

Humans are unpredictable, and roadway systems are more complex than they appear. Even though there are myriad combinations of unpredictable human behaviours playing out daily on the streets of our cities, there are certain patterns and habits that emerge and that you can come to expect given various everyday circumstances. That said, you should never take any situation for granted because things can change in an instant, and the situation might not be what it seems.

As you learn to read and anticipate these types of common movements in the road, you'll start to gain confidence and know when and how to move based on your precise position and the variables in play.

SPEED

The best, or "proper," speed is a subjective thing when it comes to bikes in the city. Some people make it a mission to keep up with motor vehicles, while others are happy just cruising along at their natural steady pace. Technically, we are obliged to ride at or below the posted speed limits — rarely an issue for most riders, though occasionally so when it comes to posted speeds on shared park paths. Average urban cyclists tend to travel between 10 and 15 km/h (6–9 mph), depending on the time of day and route selected.

Many people prefer to take the slow and steady approach, and Vélo Québec's vice-president of development and public affairs, Jean-François Pronovost, is one of them: "Bicycling and walking are for me the two most interesting and efficient ways to move in the city even though they are totally different and give totally different experiences. I am a 'slow vélo' disciple, which doesn't mean that I'm only moving slowly. I see the bicycle as an extension of the act of walking. I like to go fast enough and slow enough to be able to appreciate the environment, look at the people and anticipate emergency situations. It is my way to be cool and relaxed on a bicycle."

QUICK START GUIDE: THE BASICS

So you're ready to head out on the road. If nothing else, be sure to read the following points before you start rolling. This stuff is the bare minimum that you should know if you're going to be part of traffic on a bicycle. You'll often find yourself in roadway scenarios that you're unfamiliar with in terms of which way to go, what the signage means, and where you belong. If something seems too risky, you can always get off and walk your bike past the issue. Until you've gained confidence to know when you can claim your space and do so safely, it is often better to yield and proceed when possible. That said, if you've decided to either wait or go, don't change your mind — commit to your decision to avoid sending mixed signals and a potential collision.

1. Obey All Local Traffic Laws

When using the road, cyclists share the same rights and responsibilities as motorists. A bike is considered a vehicle, and a cyclist must obey all traffic signs and signals (though there are some circumstantial exceptions that vary by municipal or provincial/state law). If you don't have a driver's licence, you may want to pick up a driver's education manual and learn the rules of the road as they apply in your province or state.

Stop at all stop signs and red lights, unless you live in Idaho, now famous amongst cyclists for the "Idaho Stop." This law, named after the original law passed by the state of Idaho in 1982, lets cyclists treat stop signs as yield signs, which means they don't have to come to a full stop, and treat red lights as stop signs.

Although the Idaho Stop is not law in any Canadian or American cities outside that state, it is gaining popularity amongst riders — some cities, such as Winnipeg, are considering implementing the Idaho Stop, and it may become more widespread in the future. In the meantime, stop at stop signs or risk a fine: In Vancouver, for example, cyclists can be fined $167 for failing to stop as directed.

2. Keep to the Right, Except to Pass, Most of the Time . . .

Ride in the same direction as the rest of the traffic and in a straight line. In some cities, bike lanes are provided for cyclists at the side of the road, usually on the right. The majority of city streets require you to ride in the curb lane (the lane next to the sidewalk or curb) or as far to the right as practicable. So although you want to stay to the right, you also want to avoid hazards like sewer grates and debris. The general rule is to ride 1 metre (3 feet) away from the curb (or from parked cars) to avoid common urban hazards. This may at times decrease the amount of space between you and a passing motor vehicle, so use your discretion.

Pass in much the same way motorists do: Look over your left shoulder for oncoming traffic, signal left (more on this later), move into the left lane, and then pass. (If passing another cyclist, however, you can likely do so without changing lanes.) In general, pass moving cars — for example, one slowing to find on-street parking or making a right turn — on the left, ideally allowing 1 metre (3 feet) of clearance. Motorists expect you to pass on the left and are more likely to be aware of your presence if you do so. If a car is speeding up as you're trying to pass, stay in your lane, reduce your speed, wait for them to move along, and then merge back into the right lane. There is an exception to this rule, though: Never pass a vehicle on the side to which it's turning.

In general, avoid passing anyone on the right, buses and large trucks in particular. In most cities, passing on the right is illegal, and even in areas where it's allowed it's always dangerous. Some cities, like Vancouver, do allow passing on the right under certain circumstances, such as when travelling in a bike lane or when the vehicle ahead is turning left. More often than not, on a roadway without bike lanes or cycle tracks, cyclists will be sharing the curb lane with drivers. If traffic is heavy, cyclists will often be moving faster than the cars in their lane and will pass cars along the right side, between the car and the curb. That's where the whole "don't pass on the right" thing gets a bit confusing.

Cyclists riding in traffic may get tempted to squeeze through by weaving in and out between lined up cars to avoid the wait. As a rule, don't do it: Either stay to the right and pass where there is room between traffic and the curb, or just wait out the traffic like other vehicles. You can always get off your bike and walk along the sidewalk until you are past a traffic jam (and sometimes you'll still be beating traffic!). In cities like Chicago, where squeezing between cars isn't illegal (though still not recommended), impatient cyclists must watch out for car doors that can open at any time, pedestrians weaving in between traffic, and cars jutting into traffic jam openings.

As you ride around various obstacles, remember that your body tends to naturally drift toward what you are looking at. With that in mind, be sure to look toward where you want to go, rather than at the obstacle you're navigating past. For example, rather than looking at a car's mirror, look past it toward the clear space beyond.

3. Hold Your Line

The simple act of riding in a straight line is actually a really important component of city riding. Given that we're expected to ride as far to the right as possible on regular roadways, our inclination is to move back over to the right after going around obstacles and parked cars in particular. But this takes you out of the line of sight of those coming up behind you, which makes you less safe, not more. Sudden jerky movements made by riders, like when they pop back out from between parked cars, tend to freak out drivers and other cyclists. Try to ride smoothly and in a predictable straight line to communicate to other road users that you know what you're doing and that they can safely pass you when appropriate.

In a typical "two lanes in each direction" street

scenario, where the curb lane has parked cars, you'll want to ride 1 metre (3 feet), where possible, away from the parked cars and hold your roadway position even when a gap opens up on your right, between those parked cars. When the row of parked cars ends, such as when approaching an intersection, you can move to the right at this point or maintain a centre or left lane position if the parking continues in the next block. Be mindful, however, of cars wanting to turn right — you can move left enough to allow them room to pass or hold your position and let them wait as they would behind a car. Maintaining this position means that you'll be in the right spot as you approach the upcoming parked cars. Establishing and confidently maintaining the space you need to feel safe in any given roadway situation will allow other road users to see and understand how to interact with you. As Étienne Roy-Corbeil, owner of Dumoulin Bicyclettes in Montreal, points out, claiming your space is both safe and a political statement: "Not only are you taking a stand in favour of the bicycle as a legitimate means of getting around town, but you are most of all making it easy for people around you to drive/walk/cycle."

4. Take the Lane When Necessary

In most North American cities, cyclists are permitted to

"take the lane" as needed for safety by riding outside of the usual 1 metre (3 feet) curb zone on the right side of the road. Taking the lane means shifting position to the centre of the lane rather than remaining on the far right. In this position, there is no passing space for a motorist to overtake you in the same lane.

It's generally advisable and safest to take the lane when riding at the same speed as traffic or when you're avoiding potholes, grates, the doors of parked cars, construction zones, and other obstacles. Some curb lanes are also too narrow to share with passing motor vehicles, so feel free to take the lane in this case as well. Signal your intention prior to changing lane positions, and do so when there is a safe gap. Remember, it's your right to do this as needed for safety, so try not to let drivers intimidate you into moving over if you need the full lane. Move back to the right only when it's safe for you to do so.

5. Communicate Clearly

Communication and predictable riding are the best ways to stay safe while riding a bike. Making **eye contact** with pedestrians in your path and drivers at intersections or along your route is enormously helpful. Not only does it allow you to make sure you've been seen, but it also humanizes you to the person who sees

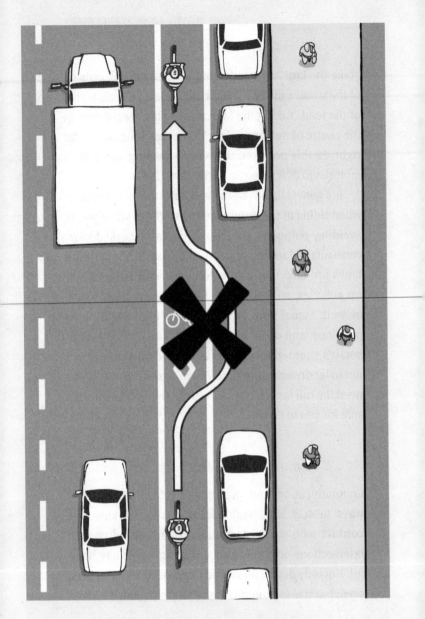

DON'T weave out of the line of sight of other road users

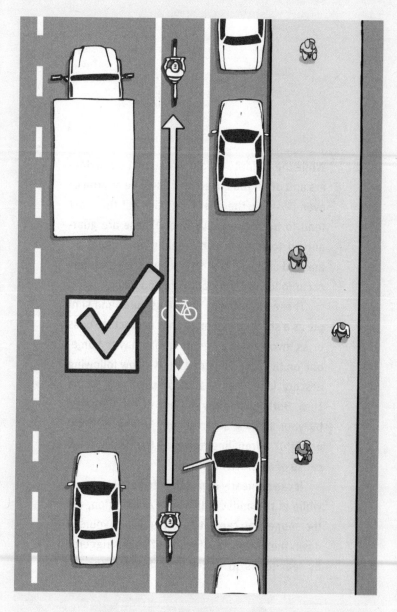

DO ride in a predictable straight line

DEALING WITH A NEGATIVE INTERACTION

While the majority of your interactions with drivers and other road users will likely be neutral or even positive, the ones that stick out the most tend to be the negative ones. These are guaranteed to happen occasionally, and you'd be amazed at the kind of stress response that may occur following a threat to life and limb.

These interactions can be as quick and simple as a shouted expletive after a too-close pass or as involved as a shouting match with someone on the other side of a car window following a scary lane change that pressed you to the curb. Both exchanges will have been triggered by your body's automatically engaged "fight or flight" adrenaline response that kicks in because of a perceived threat.

It can be nearly impossible to keep your cool while in the midst of this type of situation, but the sooner you can get past it and calm yourself down the better. This feeling of anger triggered by fear tends to linger, unfortunately, so it's really a mind over matter type thing that you need to be aware of and take steps to handle. Since you never know whom you're dealing with, it's usually better not to get into an argument in the street or touch someone's vehicle on purpose — it could prove dangerous.

you. I sometimes like to throw in a wave if I'm not entirely certain I've been seen — left-hand turners who might be more focused on cars and pedestrians, for example, often get a little wave hello from me.

Never underestimate the power of a simple smile and a wave. Acknowledging another human, just because you've seen them or because you appreciate them giving you the right of way, will almost always be well received.

Signal your intentions to drivers, pedestrians, and other cyclists using hand signals whenever you change lanes, turn, or slow or stop somewhere other than at a controlled intersection. If possible, make your signal continuously for roughly 30 metres (100 feet) before you manoeuvre. If, however, you're stopped at an intersection in a left-turn lane, for example, you don't need to keep signalling while waiting for the green since being in a dedicated turn lane helps indicate your intention. Signal again just before the light changes in your favour for extra clarity. Avoid changing lanes abruptly as drivers may not notice a quickly flashed signal. Once you've made sure the way is clear, and signalled, it's preferable to put both hands back on the handlebars so that you have full control of your bike while you manoeuvre. The main point of using hand signals is to let those around you know what you're going to do — use your best judgment in each scenario you encounter.

There are only four basic signals you need to know. When turning to the left, extend your left arm straight out to the side. To indicate a right turn, there are two options: Extend your left arm with your elbow bent and your forearm and hand pointed up, or extend your right arm out to the side. To signal stopping or slowing down, point your left arm out with your elbow bent and your arm and hand pointed down. To signal when moving within your lane, use the appropriate hand to point over and down at a 45-degree angle to the position where you plan to move.

Before you enter the roadway to start riding, turn, pass, or change lanes, be sure to **shoulder check**. Looking back over your (usually left) shoulder helps

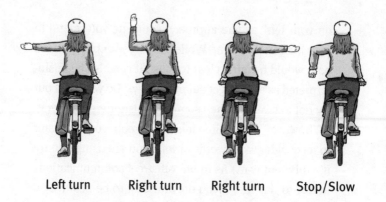

| Left turn | Right turn | Right turn | Stop/Slow |

you move left or right more safely. The trick is to do it quickly but smoothly so that you can get your eyes back on the road ahead and avoid making your bike swerve when you turn your head. It gets easier with practice, and you'll end up doing it quite often. You want to see as much as you can when you look back, so look back and away, as opposed to back and down. Rear-view mirrors that attach to your helmet or handlebar can also help you see what's coming up from behind, but these should not be used exclusively — you must always check your blind spot.

Bells and horns are effective (and usually legally required) tools to signal your presence to pedestrians, particularly on shared bike paths where joggers and dog walkers might not be aware of bikes coming around bends, or to give notice to a driver opening their door.

Your voice is also a valuable tool. Saying, "Passing

on your left" as you approach someone you intend to pass is short and clear. While dinging your bell before a pass would be fairly clear to most, it can also be misinterpreted as a "hey, get out of my way." Do your best but try not to sweat it when someone misunderstands you. (If, however, you're often misunderstood, you may want to reconsider what words or tone you are using and try it a different way.) As in our off-street communications in day-to-day life, if you do your best to be positive on the road, you're more likely to get positivity back.

6. Intersections

While they are an everyday part of urban cycling, intersections are the busiest parts of any city and where the majority of collisions occur between all road users. Always approach intersections carefully, be extra alert to what is happening in all directions, and remain visible at all times by avoiding blind spots where drivers can't see you and making eye contact with drivers and pedestrians. Watch for right turn signals and stay clear of turning vehicles, large trucks, and buses in particular. As you approach intersections, be ready to stop abruptly or take evasive action.

When approaching a red light, most riders will proceed along the curb to the right of the lineup of stopped motor vehicles. This can be a tight squeeze, so if there's

Like many experienced riders, Cory Sutela, current president of Medicine Wheel Trail Advocates, is often asked "Isn't it dangerous to commute by bike?" Here are his rules to stay alive:

1. "Go when it's safe, not when you have the right of way. I pretend that riding is a game and that all of the cars are trying to hit me. It's my role in the game to make this impossible. I don't ever pull in front of a car without making eye contact with the driver.

2. Ride predictably. In truth, cars generally aren't trying to hit you and might even be trying to avoid you. Make it easy for them (and reduce their stress about bikes) by riding smoothly, signalling your intentions, and avoiding sudden changes of direction.

3. Play the odds. Find a route that minimizes your time on high-speed and high-volume roads, even if it takes a little longer."

not enough room to advance to the front of the line, wait your turn behind the cars.

Cyclists **going straight** through an intersection are generally permitted to occupy the entire lane if doing so is the safest way to proceed, but be aware of aggressive drivers who want to jump ahead. If an intersection has multiple lanes, make sure you choose your lane and stay in it; otherwise you risk getting cut off by motorists. If you are going straight through intersections, don't stop and wait in the right-turn-only lanes. Instead, signal and merge to the rightmost through lane and proceed forward.

Now on to the dreaded left turn. For bicyclists, there are two basic types of turns: vehicular style and pedestrian or perimeter style.

In a **vehicular-style left turn**, when approaching an intersection, be sure to shoulder check for a gap in traffic, signal your intention to turn, and move to the centre-left of the lane or the left-turn lane, when clear. You may need to slow down. Be sure to yield to oncoming cars before turning, and watch for pedestrians in the crosswalk — don't cross a lane of oncoming traffic unless there is enough of a gap in the pedestrian crosswalk for you to safely get through. Complete your turn like any other vehicle by moving into the right lane after you turn. Be sure to shoulder check again before changing lanes. Never make a left turn from the far-right side of the road.

For a **pedestrian- or perimeter-style left turn**, when approaching an intersection on a green light, cycle straight through to the far-right corner and pull over in front of the crosswalk, out of the flow of traffic. Dismount, move onto the sidewalk to wait for the light, and walk your bike across the street when the light changes. If you arrive at a red light, dismount at the white line and walk with the light across the intersection. When the light changes, walk across again and then get back on your bike and continue on your way.

A popular variation of the pedestrian-style left turn is the **90-degree** or **inverted-L turn**. To do this type of turn, when you arrive at a green light, ride straight through the intersection to the far-right corner and position your bike in the new forward direction as if you were a part of traffic from the oncoming right side of the intersection. Yield to oncoming traffic, stay out of the way of pedestrians trying to cross, watch for right-turning vehicles, and wait for the green light to ride your bike through the intersection in the new direction of travel.

Similar to any other vehicle, when **turning right**, do so from the rightmost lane, use your signal, and be sure to yield to any pedestrians to your right. Be alert and watch out for other vehicles that may not see you. Use extra caution when passing to the right of cars on

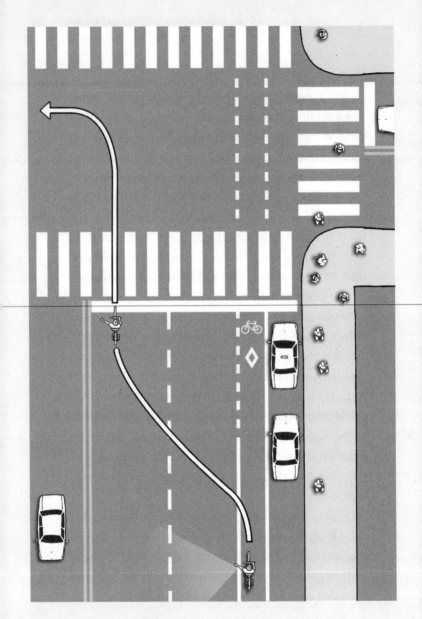

Vehicular-style left turn

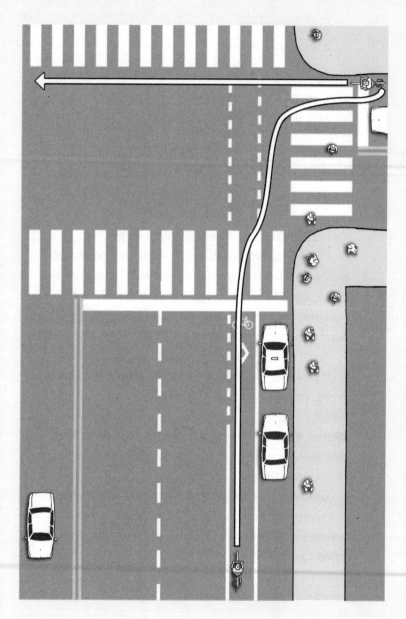

90-degree or inverted-L left turn

the approach to intersections — you'll be in drivers' blind spots, and they may be planning to turn with or without properly signalling. Stay on the lookout for right-turning cars whether or not they use their turn signals. Only pass to the right of right-turning cars if they have clearly stopped to wait for bikes and pedestrians to cross. If they've begun to turn across your path, either stop and wait until they've completed the turn or shoulder check and pass on their left.

In general, cyclists shouldn't enter an intersection on a yellow light. Yellow lights are timed for motor vehicles, not bikes, and cyclists entering the yellow light zone run the risk of being hit by drivers making left-hand turns on the yellow.

You'll also see many riders, and pedestrians, who start crossing the street before their light has turned green. Proceeding before the light has turned green is illegal — and it can be deadly. Before entering an intersection, even with a fresh green light, be sure to check that there are no straggling pedestrians or speeding cars approaching in either direction.

One final note about intersections: Drivers are used to moving along as quickly as possible within the context of the roadway and then stepping on the brakes when they hit a light. This is not an ideal technique while on a bicycle. By slowing down your pace on your approach to a red light, shifting your gears accordingly,

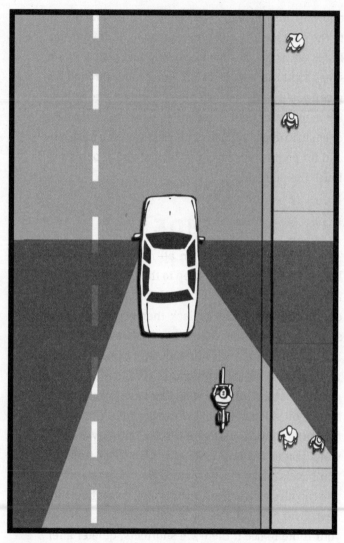

You are invisible to a driver when in their blindspot

and watching the light, you can often time your arrival to the intersection with a new green light. If your timing is off, come to a complete stop and wait for your green light. As always, before proceeding through the green you'll want to watch for oncoming traffic turning left across your path, someone coming from your right or left who might be trying to speed through a fresh red, and for pedestrians who may be inattentive or slow to finish their crossing.

WHERE TO RIDE

As a cyclist you can ride on all roads, except some highways, as long as you keep to the right (remembering the exceptions we discussed earlier), but a city's cycling infrastructure (or lack thereof) often means some routes are safer than others. When you're starting out, planning your route ahead of time can help you navigate the city safely and confidently. If your goal is to start riding to work, for example, map out a route on side streets and with bike lanes that you're comfortable with, and give it a try on the weekend, when you're not in a rush and there's less traffic. If you have a place to safely store your bike overnight, you can also ride to work one day and ride it home the next. Over time you can try out different variations on your route to see if there are shortcuts, quieter alternatives to busy roads, better infrastructure options, and the like. It's nice to change up the scenery once in a while too, and riding on low-traffic routes can also decrease your exposure to motor-vehicle-related air pollution.

As you get comfortable, and even once you are, set aside more time than you think you need; your trip is bound to be more pleasant and safer. "For the past few years I've been taking the advice I wish I could give drivers. I relax," says Todd Tyrtle, a regulatory compliance consultant from Vermont. "I'm not attached to getting somewhere as fast as my bike can get me there. Given a choice between an arterial where I might be able to manage (30 km/h [18 mph]), fighting traffic the whole way, or a parallel laneway or residential street where I average (20 km/h [12 mph]) I almost always take the laneway. What does this mean when I get to the next major street? Sometimes it means simply waiting a bit longer for a gap so I can safely cross. Sometimes, if it's very busy, it means making a quick right turn, crossing at a light and doubling back. Is this slower? Absolutely. It's still faster than walking or transit, and it's meant that the number of near-misses and driver conflicts I've experienced since making these changes has decreased from almost daily to near zero. For now I'm taking it slower and settling for getting happily across town — which is really what I ride for in the first place."

Many cities have bike-specific route maps that show you where there are bike lanes, paths, or signed routes. Your municipal transportation department or bike advocacy organization may have resources like this to help you find a safe route. Google Maps has been adding bike-specific options, and there's also a great route-planning website for many large cities in North America, Australia, and Europe called Ride the City. But, notes Clarence Eckerson Jr., director of Streetfilms, "Don't get worried about getting a little lost during your rides — especially when you have a time buffer. I've discovered more beautiful and unique places completely by chance, some only a block or two off my normal commute. Many times recommended bike routes are most direct but not the most picturesque and certainly not the most rewarding for the soul."

When you're starting to cycle, though, designated bike routes can help keep you safe. According to a 2012 study by the University of British Columbia (UBC), route types associated with a reduced risk for bike riders include cycle tracks (physically separated bike lanes), painted bike lanes, signed bike routes, minor streets, and bike paths.

UBC researcher Kay Teschke notes, "In North America, many people are fearful that it isn't safe and that deters cycling. Bicycling is actually similar in safety to walking. And evidence shows that its health benefits far outweigh any injury risks. Even so, there are ways to prevent cycling injuries. Our research shows that bike routes make a huge difference." Route types that were associated with increased injury risk included major streets without bike facilities, sidewalks, and multi-use paths.

To help you identify cyclist-friendly zones in your area, I've described some of the most common and provided some tips on how to negotiate them. For more information, check the links in the Resource Guide section.

Bike Lanes

Designed specifically for bike traffic, the roughly 1.5 metre (5 feet) lanes are painted onto the roadway, most often next to the curb or parking lane, and are usually marked by a white lane line with white bike and diamond symbols within the lane. Some bike lanes, such as those in New York, also include a painted buffer line to better separate bicyclists from other moving vehicles. Taking a lead from some European cities, some cities use green or blue paint within the lanes and where the lanes cross intersections to add even greater visibility.

If there is a bike lane, you're expected to use it,

although in most cities, such as San Francisco and Washington, D.C., cyclists may leave bike lanes and ride in regular traffic lanes if doing so makes them feel safer (or when there's no choice because someone is parked in the lane). When riding in a bike lane, follow the rules of the road and obey bike-specific signage, symbols, and signals if present. Listen for other cyclists who may want to pass you within the lane, and if you want to pass, shoulder check and use your bell and your voice as you approach.

Cars aren't supposed to stop or park in dedicated bike facilities, but cars, taxis, and quite often delivery trucks are unfortunately a daily sight in most bike lanes. If you see a motor vehicle in your path, give yourself ample time and space to merge left into a gap in traffic. Slow down if you need to in order to time your merge. Shoulder check, signal your intention, shoulder check again, and move left when it's safe to do so. The majority of drivers will see that your path is blocked and expect you to change lanes to get around the obstacle. Move back into your bike lane once the path is clear.

Some painted bike lanes position cyclists next to parked cars and right in the dreaded door zone, where an opening car door can hit you. Don't let the "safety" of the bike lane lull you into a false sense of security. To avoid getting doored, you need to remain vigilant and ride 1 metre (3 feet), or at least an arm's length, away from parked cars whenever possible, even in a bike lane.

Bike Paths

Bike paths, found off-road, are usually shared routes that are also used by pedestrians, joggers, skaters, kids, dogs, and even sometimes horseback riders. These will sometimes have a centre line similar to roadways. Calgary has an extensive bike path system known as Multi-User Pathways (MUPs) that goes both through and around the city.

When riding on bike paths, cyclists should keep to the right side, even when riding in pairs, except when passing. Always obey the posted bicycle speed limits, and if you need to stop, signal then move off the pathway to avoid collisions. As in regular on-street traffic, remain vigilant about what is happening around you, be careful about blind spots (in particular when coming around a bend), signal your intentions, and anticipate the movements of those you are sharing the path with. Slow down, pass others with care, and alert people you are overtaking with your bell or by saying "passing on your left." Always watch for dogs (and outstretched leashes) and small children who are less predictable — approach and pass slowly and with extra caution.

Shared Lanes

Shared lanes, or "sharrows," are street lanes shared by bicyclists and motorists that are marked by bike symbols and chevrons as well as posted signs. But wait, isn't every lane a "shared lane," you might ask? These bike-specific symbols are usually located on roads too narrow for bike lanes but that have enough bike traffic to warrant a visual reminder for road users to share the space. Sharrows are usually located in the curb lane, where they are applied to the road far enough away

from the curb to prevent cyclists from either colliding with car doors or riding in the space where debris gathers at the road's edge. Sharrows can also be located in the middle of a street lane. In narrower lanes, less than 4 metres (13 feet) wide, cyclists and motorists travel in a single file sharrow line for safety. The pointed end of the chevron indicates the path that a cyclist should follow. Chevrons and sharrows can also be used to indicate a merge zone, and where a bike lane crosses an intersection — the line of the bike lane stops, but the sharrows show the direction and area of travel where cyclists will cross.

Sadly, shared lanes don't offer any real protection to the rider, so remain aware of passing cars and other hazards and be prepared to slow down, stop, or change lanes at short notice.

Bike Boxes

Several North American cities, such as Edmonton, Portland, and Ottawa, have bike boxes located at some intersections. Bike boxes are large, painted (often green) squares with white bike symbols inside them. They are used at intersections to designate a space for cyclists to wait at red lights and are paired with right-turn-on-red restrictions. Some bike boxes are only at the head of the curb lane and allow cyclists a spot to

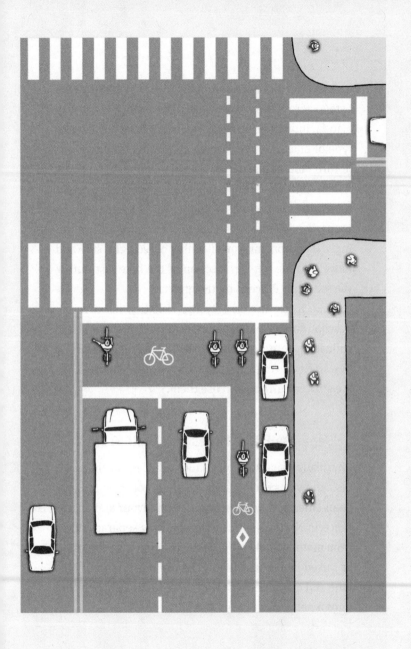

gather at the light in addition to lining up, while others extend across the whole width of both lanes in order to also facilitate left turns by cyclists. When inside each type of bike box, cyclists can go through intersections or turn first, before cars.

On a green-light approach for a left turn where a turn-lane bike box exists, change lanes so that you are properly positioned for a left turn and proceed accordingly. If approaching on an amber or red light, stop and move into the left-turn section of the bike box during the red light. Proceed on the green.

Bike boxes increase cyclist visibility, improve pedestrian safety, and decrease instances of "right hook" collisions during green lights, but they are relatively new in North America, and so drivers and cyclists alike are still learning how to use them.

Separated Bike Lanes and Cycle Tracks

Physically separated bike lanes adjacent to the road, also known as cycle tracks, are quite common in European cities and just starting to gain favour and acceptance in North America. Because they separate riders from motor vehicle traffic through some type of barrier, or raised lane, these tend to be the safest form of bike lane and one of the best ways to get more people riding once a network has been established.

Separated bike lanes are almost always accompanied by bike-specific signage and signals at intersections. Look for these and obey the directions provided when crossing or turning. Always watch for pedestrians in these lanes, since they often encroach, and be vigilant when crossing or re-entering regular traffic lanes.

Contraflow Bike Lanes

A contraflow bike lane allows bicycles to legally ride in the opposite direction on an otherwise one-way street. On my street, for example, all vehicles can travel southbound, but only bicycles can travel northbound. There is bike-specific signage at intersections as well as on-pavement white bicycle symbols and arrows indicating the direction of travel. Because it is separating opposing traffic, the painted lane line of a contraflow lane is yellow, like the centre lines on roadways. This type of lane is still fairly rare, and to date they have been used mainly to connect busy bike routes along quieter residential streets. As per regular painted bike lanes, motorists tend to park in them. Use extra caution to avoid oncoming vehicles when proceeding around cars parked in this type of lane. It may be safer to walk your bike around the obstacle on the sidewalk, rather than move into oncoming traffic.

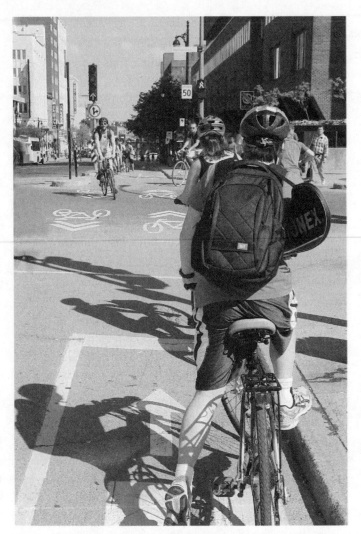

Separated, bi-directional cycle track

Bi-directional Bike Lanes

These on-street lanes are usually the width of a regular traffic lane but physically separated from motor vehicles. They have a centre line and allow bikes to travel in either direction, which is indicated by arrows within both parts of the lane. Extra caution should be used when passing to ensure you have enough time and space to safely avoid oncoming riders.

Signed Bike Routes/Bicycle Boulevards

Local transportation departments often designate quiet residential or side streets with lower volumes of traffic as preferred bicycle routes. They are marked by signage that can sometimes have specific route numbers and often provide a more bike-friendly route that follows busier main street corridors. Other than the signage, they rarely have additional on-street bike infrastructure, though a route may include a street with an existing bike lane.

Wrong-way Riding

While it's always advisable (and legally mandated) to ride in the same direction as the traffic you're part of, there are some occasions, due to the nature of bicycles,

TRIGGERING THE LIGHTS AT INTERSECTIONS BY BIKE

Traffic lights at smaller intersections, or in dedicated turn lanes, are quite often triggered by vehicles as they roll over electrically charged wires that have been embedded in the roadway. Some cities have intersections with a spot that is marked to show bicycles where they should stop to trigger the light to change. For example, Toronto has three white dots in a line. While not all cities have gotten this far, there are an increasing number of bike-specific signals and buttons placed in reach of riders at intersections.

when riding against traffic on smaller residential side streets is safer (than being on a major roadway) or faster or more direct (than taking a long detour), or both. Never ride against the flow of city traffic on main streets or in bike lanes.

If you must ride the wrong way on a one-way residential street, there are ways to do it more safely:

◊ Always obey stop signs or signals, even if there are none specific to you at intersections because they're positioned for traffic coming in the other direction.

◊ Glve right of way to oncoming drivers, in particular at narrow points in the road. Stop and put your foot down so that they know they can safely pass you.

◊ Cede right of way to pedestrians and watch for them — they won't be looking in your direction when checking for oncoming traffic.

◊ If there is on-street parking on only one side, ride on the side without parking so that you are more visible to oncoming drivers and cyclists.

◊ If there is heavy oncoming traffic, dismount and walk your bike on the sidewalk until you are back on a street where you can ride in the right direction.

◊ Always use lights at night so that drivers, pedestrians, and fellow riders can see you.

Sidewalks, Crosswalks, and Shared Pedestrian Areas

Sidewalks are for pedestrians, and in many larger North American cities it's illegal to ride on sidewalks. Some cities allow it, though only in certain areas or for riders up to a certain age.

In places where the roadway is unsafe and there is minimal pedestrian traffic, sidewalk riding is sometimes the only safe option. But be warned: drivers aren't looking out for cyclists in pedestrian spaces. One of the most common collisions to occur between bike riders and motor vehicles is at an intersection or driveway where a bike is crossing from the sidewalk, rather than in the roadway with the rest of traffic.

If concern for your safety means you must occasionally ride on the sidewalk, slow way down and always give right of way to any pedestrian you encounter. Better yet, as you approach someone who is walking, get off your bike and walk it past them for maximum safety and consideration. I'll never forget the recent story of a 15-year-old boy who was riding on the sidewalk along a major high-speed roadway in his suburban neighbourhood. Although this was really the safest, and legal, place for him to ride, tragedy still struck when he encountered a local senior making her way to nearby shops. According to the police report, they both tried to avoid each other but moved to the same side at the same time. He unintentionally knocked her down and she fell straight back, hitting her head. She died a short

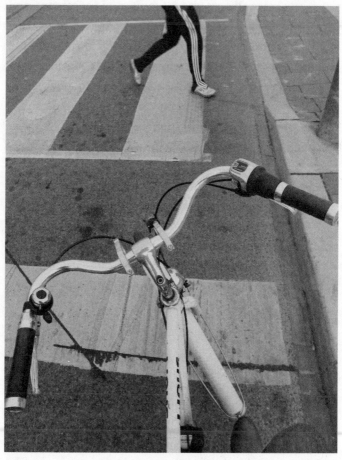

Stopping position at intersections

time later in hospital from her injury. Sidewalks are pedestrian territory — as a visitor, and some might say trespasser, it's your job to stay clear.

Crosswalks are also the territory of pedestrians, and if you're approaching or passing across a crosswalk by bike, always yield to pedestrians. When stopping at a red light, always stop behind the white line and leave the crosswalk clear for pedestrians. Stopping inside the crosswalk is basically the same thing as someone parking in the bike lane — not cool. When crossing with pedestrians at a crosswalk, you should walk your bike unless a local bylaw and corresponding on-street markings permit you to ride through. Some cities, like Vancouver, have what are called "crossbikes," or "elephants' feet": crosswalks that allow cyclists to ride across at the same time as pedestrians in a designated space. These shared crosswalks usually have bike-specific markings running along the sides.

NEGOTIATING URBAN OBSTACLES

While many people are confident riders on country roads or bike paths, the challenges presented by the city can be understandably nervous-making. But forewarned is forearmed, and I've put together advice to help you handle the next city bus, aggressive taxi, or the threat of dooring. Remember to take the time to assess the scenario — sometimes these hazards call for a quick circumvention or are best avoided by slowing or stopping to wait it out.

Hills

For your average everyday rider, hills mean pleasure and pain — we love the thrill of riding down them, but heading up a hill can be torture. The nice thing about hills is that the more you ride them, the stronger you get, and the easier they are to conquer.

Your best bet is slow and steady, often in the lowest gear. As you begin the start of a climb and lose the momentum you might have brought into it, shift down to your lowest, or near lowest, gear so that pedalling is easier. Struggling and straining up a hill in a high gear is a sure way to make you avoid hills in the future. This is what gears are made for: low for climbs and starting from a stop, high for descents, and shifting up and down as needed through all situations that arise on your ride. If you need extra power, you can try getting off your saddle and pedalling in a standing position. There's no shame in walking part way if you can't keep pedalling, and sometimes this is a safer option than continuing to push yourself too hard.

While riding downhill stay balanced, use both brakes

to control your speed relative to conditions, traffic, and roadway hazards, and be cautious about how much speed you have when approaching and passing through intersections. You want to maintain the ability to slow, stop, or manoeuvre safely if something crosses your path.

On-street Parking

Drivers who are looking for on-street parking are quite obvious — they tend to slow down, hesitate, move closer to the parked cars — but as they search for an elusive parking space, you may not be so obvious to them. Cars leaving on-street parking often don't think to look for bikes, so watch for drivers, brake lights, turn signals, or other signs of life in parked cars.

The other big threat with on-street parking is dooring, a.k.a. the "door prize" (that no one ever wants to receive), which is when a driver opens the door into traffic and a cyclist is then either hit by, or collides with, that door. Taxi passengers are quite likely the second-greatest cause of dooring incidents, and these can happen just about anywhere, and on either side of the taxi, since they often stop mid-block, mid-lane, at intersections, or anywhere at all really. Also watch for regular cars dropping off passengers mid-block or at corners.

Avoiding a dooring incident requires constant vigilance on the part of bike riders and on the part of people exiting motor vehicles. It takes place in an instant, and the results can be anywhere from minor to deadly. Anytime you are passing parked or stopped motor vehicles, there is a chance of a door opening on the driver or passenger side — always be on the lookout and try to ride 1 metre (3 feet) away from parked or stopped cars.

Construction Zones

Construction zones are a big part of city life, and not just on-street construction — fences around new buildings often push out into the roadway for part of the construction period. These hot spots mean a change in roadway condition and also the flow of traffic before, through, and after the construction zone. Depending on the stage of construction, there may be significant debris in the roadway, and there are often trucks or other heavy machinery galore. Always obey police or construction crews that are directing traffic to accommodate these trucks — the delay will only be for a moment or two, and it's not worth trying to squeeze through.

As you approach a construction site, the lane you're in may narrow or end completely. Shoulder check, signal, and then merge when you're able. When the roadway opens back up after a construction zone, drivers try to make up lost time. Keep an eye on their speed, and, as soon as you are able, move back to your regular riding position on the right side of the curb lane.

Trucks, Buses, and Large Motor Vehicles

These large vehicles are very common on the road and should be treated with extra caution. This is not an enemy you want to engage; in fact, you generally want to keep your distance and always give them right of way. These vehicles may be driven by professionals, but even professionals make mistakes, like not signalling a turn. Drivers of these large vehicles also have big blind spots in front, in back, and on the sides.

Always watch for their signals and stay well back so that you can respond in time to a change in lane position, turn, or reduction in speed. Avoid riding beside a truck or bus — if need be, slow down and allow them to pass you.

If you end up beside a bus or truck at a light because they've come up from behind, don't assume this means they have seen you. To be extra safe, you could simply move onto the sidewalk and wait until they clear on the green. This is always what you should do if they appear to be making a right turn. If you prefer to continue along straight (you were there first after all), pull slightly ahead into the drivers' line of vision and

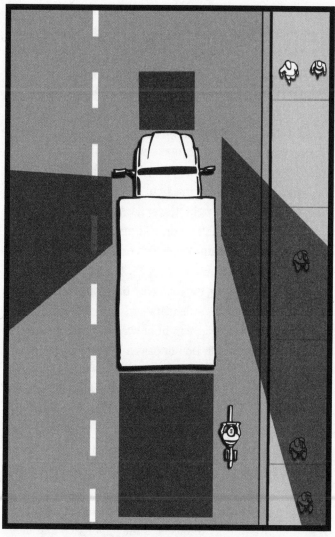

Stay back to stay safe — avoid these blindspots

make eye contact. Once you've been seen, you can then either move slightly in front of the truck and get a quick start on the light, forcing the larger vehicle to slow and change lanes to pass you, or you can shift further to the right, closer to the crosswalk, proceed slowly on the green, and then merge back into traffic once the vehicle has moved along.

Trucks and buses make wide right turns and, depending on the intersection design and traffic circumstances, also sometimes cut in very close on or over the curb to their right. Never pass a truck or bus on the right that is signalling or beginning a right-hand turn. Stay well back until they've completed the turn and gone on their way.

When sharing the road with buses and other transit vehicles, such as streetcars and light rail, you have a responsibility to give right of way to the passengers as they get on or off. Do not pass a bus that has its doors open, though you can pass to the left of a bus that is at the curb. Wait until all passengers have cleared the roadway before proceeding. School buses have stop signs attached that are deployed when students are getting on or off the bus. Just like cars, bikes are required to obey these stop signs and wait until the signs have been turned off to proceed or pass the school bus. In some cities, all other vehicles are required to yield and give priority to buses as they approach and move on from the stops along their designated routes. In any case, give these wide loads a wide berth.

Taxis

Taxis tend to follow their own version of the rules of the road and are as likely to pull a sudden U-turn as they are to pull over to the curb in front of you without checking. Passengers are equally unpredictable — they are often distracted and in a rush during the day and may be drunk at night. Expect the unexpected with taxis, keep your distance to avoid a dooring, and always ride defensively around them.

Emergency Vehicles

Fire, ambulance, and police vehicles always have priority on the road when their emergency lights and/or sirens are activated. All vehicles are required by law to pull over as far to the right as possible and stop until the emergency vehicle has passed them. Bicycles are no exception. It may sometimes be safer for you to move off the roadway entirely and onto the sidewalk — do what feels appropriate in the moment.

Traffic Circles and Roundabouts

Although these are not as common as intersections controlled by stop signs, traffic circles and round-abouts can be found in many cities as a form of traffic calming. Slow down on your approach; you don't need to stop completely if the way is clear. Look left to see if anyone is coming around the circle, and yield to vehicles already in the intersection. Enter the circle and proceed to the right. At the spot where you are planning to exit the circle, indicate your intention to turn right. Don't forget to watch for and yield to pedestrians when entering and exiting.

Darkness

Being visible to other road users on your bike at night is not only crucial to your safety and well-being, it's also a common courtesy for those around you. Street lights just aren't enough. Most cities in North America require by law that bikes have some combination of white front headlight and red rear reflectors and/or red rear light, which are widely recognized as indicators of bicycles. Headlights and rear lights generally need to be visible from a range of 100–150 metres (300–500 feet).

Some urban areas, however, such as Toronto, New York, Calgary, and Gainesville, Florida, require a headlight, rear reflector, *and* a red rear light. Other cities, including Chicago, Ottawa, Boulder, and Moncton, only require a headlight and rear reflector, although they generally encourage a red rear light as well. Check your city's rules before cycling at night, but remember it's a good idea to err on the safe side. I never ride after dark without both a front and rear light and always make sure to bring them along when heading out for the day.

Most North American cities strongly encourage additional reflectors to enhance cyclists' visibility at night. Reflectors should be added to your bike spokes and pedals, and you may even want to put reflecting tape strips, which can be found at some bike shops and hardware stores, on your helmet and clothes. Basically, the more visible you are to other vehicles the better. Lighter-coloured clothing can also help increase your visibility.

If you must travel at night through an area known to be somewhat sketchy, you are usually much safer on a bike than you would be on foot. Stay alert when in an unsafe area — consider taking the full lane so that you're away from the sidewalk, where someone could approach you. Additionally, if you end up stopped at a light, stop as far from the curb as is safe and remain aware of what is happening in all directions. If you don't feel safe stopping at a light, make a right-hand

LOCK IT OR WALK IT: DRINKING AND RIDING

While riding drunk might seem like a convenient workaround to drinking and driving, drinking impairs your ability to ride safely and greatly increases your risk of a crash or injury. If you're not in shape to ride, you can either use your bike as a walker to get you home or, if that won't work, lock up your bike (ask for help if you need it) and cab, walk, or take transit home. If you have a cell phone or something to write on, be sure to make note of where you've left your trusty steed, either by leaving yourself a voicemail, taking a photo, or scribbling the location down on paper.

turn so that you can continue moving. If there isn't much traffic, you may then be able to make a U-turn and another right-hand turn so that you can continue in your intended direction of travel. If you are being threatened and there's no oncoming traffic, you should proceed through a red light to get away.

Riding at night can be more hazardous not only because of reduced visibility, but on Friday and Saturday nights in particular, because of inebriated pedestrians and sometimes drivers. While you can come across drunk folks just about anywhere in a city, there are often entertainment districts or streets where a greater concentration of inebriated people can be expected, in particular at closing time when people start to make their way home. When the ball game lets out, for example, it might be smarter not to ride near the stadium — and the unhappy-drunk or happy-drunk fans. Be extra vigilant when watching for pedestrians coming out from between parked cars, stepping off the curb to cross mid-block, or standing in the curb lane to hail a taxi.

ROAD SURFACE CONDITIONS

When you're out on the road, there's a lot to keep an eye out for in traffic and on the sidewalk, but watching for changes in the road surface ahead of you is equally important. Remember, if a curb lane is too narrow to safely share with motorists while also avoiding roadside hazards, you are entitled to take the lane.

Debris of all types is usually found at the edge of the road — that very same space bicycles are expected to occupy. Following a heavy rain, grit, dirt, leaves, water, and garbage often accumulate near storm grates and along the edge of the curb. **Large puddles** are also best avoided since they can hide other hazards, like grates and potholes, and may be deeper than expected.

Uneven pavement, bumps and potholes in the road are the most frequent causes of a fall, crash, or damage to your wheels. Depending on your location in the road, volume of traffic, and other factors, sometimes you can safely and quickly take evasive action around the obstacle. If this isn't feasible, slow down as much as possible, stand up out of your seat, and use your arms and legs as shock absorbers to avoid a big, heavy hit.

Gravel, grit, and sand in the road are serious hazards for turns in particular. Smaller loose grit can cause you to slip on a turn made with speed, and gravel can also cause a fall by forcing you off balance. Slow down and approach with caution.

Black tar is often used to fill in cracks that develop in the roadway. During the heat of summer, these long strips can become soft and squishy. They can also catch your tires and are best avoided.

Motor oils can accumulate on the roadway during dry, hot periods and then be drawn up to the surface when it rains. If you are caught riding in a rainstorm following a long dry spell, be aware that the road surface may become slick in some places, such as where cars often park in the curb lane.

Piles of **slippery, wet autumn leaves** can take you down and hide things like grates and potholes. Try to avoid them, and use extra caution on turns in particular. (For more on riding in rain, ice, and snow, see pages 105–107.)

When possible, steer clear of **sewer covers** and other metal ground coverings. These are generally less grippy than the roadway and even more slippery when wet or snow covered.

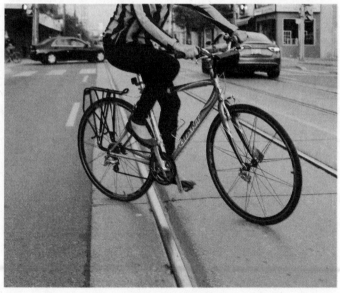

Cross railway and streetcar tracks on an angle

Railway and streetcar tracks can be dangerous if you cross at the wrong angle. Bike wheels can get stuck in or along the track or can slip sideways across the slick metal surface. Tracks become more slippery when they're wet, so be extra cautious when riding in the rain or in snowy weather. The best way to avoid getting your wheel stuck is to always cross tracks at a right angle — you want to go perpendicular, not parallel, to the track. Use the same approach for slots or cracks in the pavement and sewer grates.

Remember, if you are not comfortable riding over tracks, either because there are multiple tracks at an intersection, difficult track angles, or because of traffic, you can always pull over to the curb, get off your bike, and cross the intersection as a pedestrian.

Like any other vehicle, bicycles must obey the signs and barriers in use at a **railway crossing**. Stop and wait until the train has passed if the lights are flashing and the barrier arms are across the road. No exceptions. Anytime you are approaching and preparing to cross railway tracks, look both ways to be sure that no train is coming.

DISTRACTED CYCLING

Distracted cycling is as much a concern as distracted driving. If you must use your cell phone while on the road, pull over somewhere appropriate to answer or make a call. Texting while riding is definitely a bad idea. It only takes a moment of distraction while looking at your phone to end up in a crash. Make it a rule to never use your phone while riding. Not only will you be safer, you'll be better able to enjoy the analog simplicity of your gears and brakes, as well as that much-needed break from your digital tether.

Headphones are also generally a bad idea. In dense pedestrian and traffic-heavy cities, riders always need to be fully aware of their surroundings, and that includes being tuned into sounds like approaching cars and bikes, emergency vehicle sirens, the click or beep of an unlocking car door, the sounds of something falling off your bike, or a passing call from a fellow rider. You really need all of your senses to stay safe and alert in city traffic.

Most North American cities prohibit cyclists from wearing headphones to some degree. Cities like Montreal, Boulder, and Gainesville, Florida, prohibit the wearing of headphones completely, while other areas, including San Francisco and New York, permit cyclists to wear a headphone in one ear while keeping the other ear free to hear traffic noises. In many urban areas, there aren't specific laws regarding headphones, but pretty much every city discourages cyclists from wearing them.

Headphones may not be a great idea, but there are still great options for playing music while riding. It can be as low tech as putting your MP3 player or phone into a handlebar-mounted metal coffee mug along with a small speaker that fits into the headphone jack. The mug will keep your device safe and amplifies the sound coming out of the speaker. There are also more sophisticated systems on the market; just search online for "music player for bicycles."

BIKES ON TRANSIT

Most large North American cities (and many smaller ones) have some form of public transportation system that cyclists can make use of to increase their travel efficiency and to cover longer distances. I regularly use the subway to get uphill when I'm heading further uptown during the day and then ride home downhill.

Bikes on Buses Keep your eye out for front-mounted exterior bike racks. These racks can usually hold two bikes securely for cyclists who need to take the bus. In some instances, if bike racks are full and especially in periods outside of rush hours, some bus drivers will let cyclists bring their bikes onto the bus.

Most cities with buses that hold bikes on front-mounted racks have instructions and videos on their websites about how to properly load your bike. If you've never used a bus bike rack before, it can seem daunting — the videos are really helpful.

Bikes on Trains Cities with subway or above-ground train systems usually allow cyclists to bring their bikes aboard, although there are sometimes time-of-day restrictions against bikes, particularly during peak travel times. Check your city's local transit website for details on restrictions for bikes on trains and buses. In some cities, folding bikes are exempt from time-of-day restrictions on trains — if you're regularly taking your bike on transit, this could be a great option.

CYCLIST-ON-CYCLIST ETIQUETTE

With more people commuting by bike, the number of cyclists sharing the edge of our urban roads has been rising steadily, especially during rush hour. Simple bike etiquette can improve the ride for everyone.

◊ Signal your intentions: Don't be afraid of verbal and non-verbal communication. If you don't remember what signals to use, just point in the direction you are going to go.

◊ Shoulder check before making a move: Be sure a faster cyclist or driver isn't coming up behind you as you enter the roadway or change lane position.

◊ Don't wear headphones. These disconnect you from other road users and are a distraction.

◊ If you are about to pass, a single ding of the bell or casual and friendly "On your left" as you approach is usually well received. Always alert a rider that has been stopped at a red light that you are overtaking on a new green light.

◊ Wait until it is safe to pass: Don't endanger yourself or other riders by squeezing through when there is not enough room.

◊ If there's enough space to get through and local laws allow it, you don't have to wait in line at a red if you want to turn right, but it's usually more about the timing. If you have enough space and time to pass everyone and turn before the new green, you should use your bell to let others know you're coming. Otherwise line up and wait your turn.

◊ Tailgating is for bike races: Leave enough space, two to three bike lengths, between you and the cyclist you are following — if they stop suddenly, you need room to manoeuvre and enough space to stop.

◊ Riding the wrong way in a bike lane is not cool.

◊ Locking to someone else's bike is even less cool!

◊ As when driving, texting or talking on your phone while biking is too big of a distraction. Wait or stop and pull over onto the sidewalk.

◊ Try to be aware and accommodating of the faster and slower riders around you. We all have a preferred pace, and sometimes we're in a hurry or taking our time.

◊ With more skateboarders on the roads, and in bike lanes, you can safely treat them like you do fellow cyclists, and expect similar behaviour. Watch for runaway skateboards and do your best to avoid them.

◊ If you *must* roll through a stop sign, slow down and check that no one is coming, and that includes pedestrians and other bikes. Stop if someone's there and wait your turn.

◊ Watch when and where you spit please! The wind can make for unexpected spit showers.

◊ If you make a mistake, please apologize.

Above all, remember that it's not a race — ride predictably, try to be patient, and smile. As a general rule, in life and while riding, I like to keep in mind the lyrics of my wise friend Michael Louis Johnson, a long-time cycling activist and talented musician: "Don't do to the dude what you don't want the dude to do to you."

Patience: Any minor inconvenience is likely to last no more than a few seconds, though it may feel like longer.

TIPS FOR
ALL-WEATHER RIDING

Weather presents both physical and psychological challenges, which means that most people are fair-weather riders. That's okay, of course, but know that with the right attitude and prep, you can ride in just about any weather. Doing so is also guaranteed to make you feel like a badass. Make checking the forecast a morning ritual if it isn't already, then be sure to bring along whatever might be needed throughout the day and evening. If there's even a chance of rain, my rain poncho comes along — better safe and prepared than sorry, wet, and miserable. I also make a habit of carrying an extra top layer in spring and fall since the temperature usually dips after the sun goes down.

The tips below are general and can be adapted and supplemented as needed, based on your riding style, experience, and climate.

Sun

There's nothing quite as lovely as a beautiful sunny day for a bike ride. The sun is, however, our frenemy. So as the Australians say, "Slip! Slop! Slap!" for sun protection. Slip on a long-sleeve shirt. Slop on some sunscreen. Slap on a hat. They've also recently added

"Seek!" shade or shelter and "Slide!" on some sunglasses. Even on short rides to work, sunscreen on your face and exposed skin is advised — don't forget your ears, lips, hands, hair part, and tops of your feet. Over time, exposure adds up.

During extreme heat, it's best to slow your pace and not get your heart rate up too high. When you're riding, the breeze you create with your momentum will keep you relatively cool; it's when you stop at lights or your destination that you really notice just how hot you've become. Try to pace yourself, take it easy, and stick to shady routes when possible. Stay hydrated by bringing along a reusable water bottle that you can reach and use easily while on the go. You can buy a bottle holder for your bike ($5 to $25), and most bikes come with the mounting screws already in place for one.

When riding in the heat of summer, I always make sure to bring along a sweat rag and a paper hand fan. The sweat rag is usually a bandanna tied around my wrist or tucked in somewhere handy, so that I can dab away dripping sweat while on the move. When I arrive at my destination, and my free and natural air conditioning gets locked up with my ride, I pull out the hand fan to keep the air moving so that I can cool down more quickly. It's amazing how effective these little things are, though the fan is admittedly a bit more culturally associated with women. If your city has a Chinatown neighbourhood, this is where you'll likely be able to pick one up.

Rain

The rain, although miserable at times, need not stop you from using your bike to get around. A full rain protection kit includes a rain jacket or poncho with hood or visor, rain pants, a waterproof helmet cover, booties that slip over your shoes, and a bag or pannier to carry everything in before and after the rain. For short trips in the rain, a simple poncho or rain jacket will do. Admittedly, it took me a while to come around to the booties, but when it's really coming down hard and you've got a fair distance to cover, these can make life much more pleasant by keeping your feet happy and dry in combination with rain pants.

Rain ponchos, such as Cleverhoods, have come a long way and are more versatile, stylish, and handy than ever. On shorter rides or in a light rain, you can even ditch the rain pants since the poncho can be held out front (via the handy little thumb rings that some have) and over your handlebars, creating a tent over your lower body. This does leave you vulnerable to splashes from passing vehicles and from big puddles, but they're simple one-piece rain protection that will keep you from getting soaked through.

Visibility is poorer for everyone during a rainy ride, at night in particular. Lights, clothing, gear, and a bike with reflective surfaces and bright colours, along with extra caution, can help keep you safe in the rain, snow, and other inclement weather. Riding as though you can't be seen is a good way to stay out of harm's way. For example, if a driver won't see you making a left turn, perhaps you can opt for a pedestrian-style left turn instead (see page 61).

Fog

As with rain, maintaining high visibility with bright, reflective clothing and good front and rear lights is important; however, depending on just how dense the fog is, sometimes it's best not to ride at all in this type of weather. Even the best-lit car can be impossible to see in heavy fog, and it's not worth the risk of having someone not see you until it's too late. If you get caught out in a fog unexpectedly, turn on your lights immediately and consider walking your bike on the sidewalk with lights on until the fog dissipates or you pass beyond it.

Snow and Ice

Cold-weather riding requires more preparation and attention than riding in other types of weather, but hardy cyclists will tell you it's still worth it. Since salt can do corrosive damage to your bike frame and parts, some people have a winter "beater bike" for this purpose. Layers are your best friend and will keep you comfortable when riding in the cold. Wool in particular is important for its moisture-wicking properties. But be careful not to overdress. It may sound counterintuitive, but you're better off starting your ride a little bit chilly since you'll have warmed up within three or four minutes of starting your engine. You'll still sweat while riding, even if you're not overdressed. To avoid getting chilled, be sure to take off your layers when you arrive at your destination so that you a) don't sweat even more and further dampen your clothes, and b) you can dry out any layers that have become humid before layering up to head out again. Wet layers can cause you to become chilled.

"I am often asked how it's possible to commute in sub-zero temperatures," says Cory Sutela, test development engineer for SRAM. "My answer is always, 'I'm warmer than you are in your car.' The longer answer is, 'I have the right equipment for the conditions.' In the coldest of conditions I bring out the big guns — hiking boots on platform pedals, fleece insulating layers, burly mitts instead of gloves, snowboard helmet, ski goggles, full Gore-Tex outer layer. When it's warmer I always carry a contingency layer in my pack — balaclava, leg warmers, toe covers, and an extra lightweight riding jacket. With these I am prepared for rapid weather changes without giving up much space in the pack."

Avoid exposed skin by covering your ears (ear muffs and certain knit hats can work with helmets), hands (try combining inner gloves with outer mitts), face (with a scarf or balaclava), and eyes (with glasses or even ski goggles!). A heavy moisturizer and lip balm will also help your skin survive harsh, cold wind and weather. If you're riding with your face or nose exposed on a cold sunny day, remember to wear sunscreen on longer rides — you're still vulnerable to sunburn in the winter.

When it comes to riding on snow and ice, first and foremost, slow down and brake lightly. Unless you've invested in a pair of metal studded tires (not necessary but useful in some super wintery cities), you're more vulnerable to a wipeout in this type of slippery scenario. If you come across a patch of flat ice, such as a frozen puddle, that you are unable to ride around, remain calm and try not to tense your body. Stop pedalling, stay balanced, and roll straight over it. The worst thing to do is panic and brake or try to turn suddenly on the ice. If you've come across a stretch of roadway that is too icy to ride, or that makes you uncomfortable, you can always dismount and walk your bike until the road clears. I make a habit in the winter of testing the slipperiness of the roadway with my feet before starting a ride.

When you get to your destination, remember that you're bringing in the debris, mud, salt, rain, or snow that goes with whatever the season. Give your ride a good bounce or two to knock off excess crud before bringing it inside, and then park it on top of old newspapers, or a dedicated bike towel, to help contain the rest of the dirt and muck that will drip off your frame and wheels.

If you're just getting started riding when the weather is nice, don't think you've got to take the plunge and ride all through the winter. If cycling regularly ends up being your thing, you'll figure out what works best for you and adapt to weather conditions over time. As the League of American Bicyclists' president, Andy Clarke, suggests, "The most important advice: Get out there and try it. Don't be daunted by the need to do everything at once or solve every conceivable problem at the outset. Do what you feel comfortable doing. Once you're out there on the street, remember that most of urban cycling survival is paying attention and being conscious of your surroundings. It may sound silly, but always expect that the people around you will do the stupidest thing imaginable — and be ready for it. And, of course, be sure to take advantage of bike safety classes and resources from your local bike advocacy organization or the League's Smart Cycling program."

3

Common Cyclist Setbacks

As exhilarating and efficient as riding a bike can be, there are certainly a few setbacks that can be expected along your way to becoming a confident city cyclist. Bike theft, crashes, and traffic tickets can all seem pretty overwhelming, but they need not be insurmountable obstacles that keep you off your bike. Read on for how to avoid, and get through, the rough patches.

BIKE THEFT

Having your bike stolen is straight-up heartbreak and an all-too-common occurrence in our cities. But locking your bike properly, with a good lock, can let you rest a bit easier about your ride. Even if you're just running into a shop to buy a pack of gum, there is never a good reason to leave your bike unattended and un-locked. You can also help out others with a little bit of "neighbourhood watch" style community support: Without putting yourself in harm's way, if you notice someone messing with a bike, say something — even a joke will do.

Choose the Right Lock

It generally costs you more time and money to replace a bike than to invest in a good-quality lock, so it may be worth taking a second look at yours. Eric Kamphof of Toronto's Curbside Cycle warns, "Never buy a cheap cable lock. It's like locking your house with a screen door." I love my thick, cloth-covered Abus chain: It's super strong and gives me the flexibility to lock to more than just typical bike parking, often designed with a U-lock in mind. You may want to use two different kinds of locks, one chain and one U-lock. This tough combo makes your bike harder to steal quickly since different tools are required, and breaking two locks takes longer.

Lock It Up Tight

Pay attention to what you're locking your bike to. Is it solid and fixed to the ground? If in doubt, check for

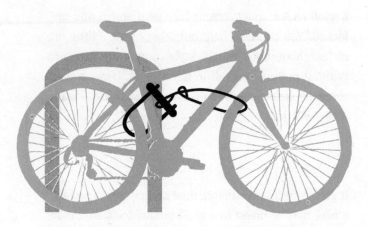

gaps where your lock might slip through, and do the wiggle test by pushing back and forth on the fence, post, or whatever to see if it's firmly secured. Avoid locking to chain-link or wooden fences, which are easy to cut through, and lock to the post part of the chain link if there are no other options. Always lock through your frame and one of your wheels (preferably the back one, where all of your gears are). If you have a rear wheel lock, use your main lock to go through the frame and front wheel. With a second lock, or a long and strong cable, you can also lock your front wheel to your frame for added security. If you're using a U-lock, the bigger a gap you leave when locking, the more likely your U-lock can be busted open with a bit of torque. Keep it tight. Locking tightly will also help prevent your bike from falling over, which could damage it or trip up pedestrians. A less conventional anti-theft strategy? Personalize your bike. I love my flower-covered basket: Aside from being pretty and making me more visible when riding, it's also a theft deterrent. "Uglification" is also an option if you've invested in a higher-end bike and want to mask its value.

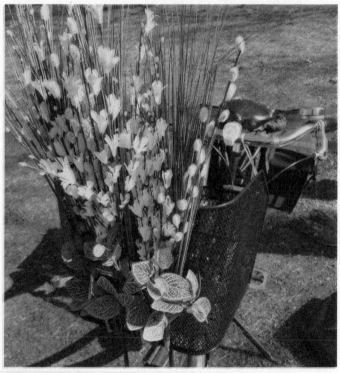

A decorated basket can help deter theft and make people smile

Common courtesy suggests that you should never lock your bike to someone else's without permission. Be particularly mindful of cables, as it's possible to catch this part of someone else's bike without noticing. You'll also want to avoid locking to private property, onto access ramps, or around small urban trees that can be damaged by your lock.

Easily removable bike parts and accessories are also easy pickings for thieves. Try to make a habit of removing your lights when you lock your bike and putting them back on when you unlock again. Unless you absolutely need them, do not use quick release on your wheels or seat post. You can buy kits ($20 to $40) to swap out the quick-release skewers for bolt skewers on your wheels and seat post. If you prefer quick release, always remember to remove one of your wheels and lock it to the frame and take your seat with you. More expensive saddles can also be secured with a seat lock fashioned out of bike chain.

In general, it's best to avoid leaving your bike outside overnight, but if you must try to leave it somewhere that is well lit, on private or semi-private property, and as securely locked as possible.

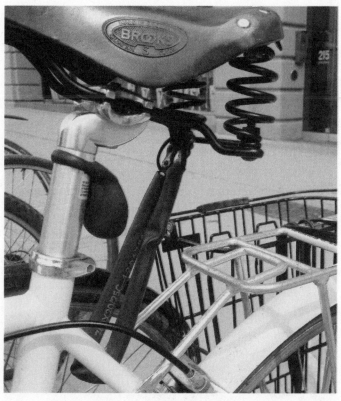

Use a piece of bike chain covered in an old tube
to lock down your seat

Keep a Record

Even if you're super careful, your ride might still go
missing, and in that case you'll want some documen-
tation. Take a photo of your bike and mark down key

identifying information such as the registration number. This is usually on the underside of the bottom bracket — flip the bike over and take a look. If your bike is stolen, you'll at least have these details handy and can prove it's yours should it be recovered.

If you're comfortable doing so, and the service exists as it does where I live, in Toronto, use these details to register your bike with your local Police Bicycle Registry service. If the police recover stolen property, they can only return it to you if your bike is in the system.

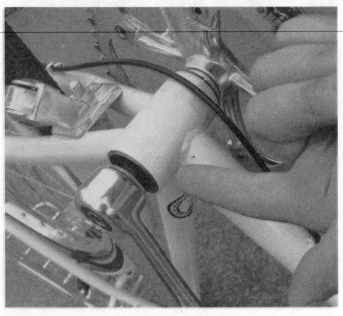

Each bike frame has a unique serial number

WHAT TO DO IF YOU'RE PULLED OVER BY THE POLICE

No one likes getting fined or ticketed, ever, for anything, but it does happen on occasion and usually serves a purpose. While cyclists used to rarely report getting ticketed, as the number of riders has grown dramatically, there's been increasing pressure on municipal police forces to be more diligent about enforcing the laws as they apply to people riding bikes.

If you don't think you did anything wrong and have some way of proving it, or at least a way to make the case, you may want to fight the ticket. You can always check in with your local cycling advocacy organization to ask for their thoughts on the matter — they may know of similar cases and have insights to share. For example, if you receive a ticket for not having bike lights or a bell, you can often get the fine waived, or at least have the amount reduced, if you present a receipt of purchase and photo evidence of said lights or bell installed on your bike.

Cycling advocates can also advise you on whether or not your ticket is written up correctly according to local traffic laws as they apply to cyclists. You'd be amazed at how often I've heard stories about tickets issued for things like not wearing a helmet in places where no mandatory helmet law actually exists. Most people — including some people who are charged with enforcing them — aren't up to date on laws, and there are many misperceptions about what is, or is not, illegal.

Once you've been stopped by police, the goal is to minimize the damage, and above all avoid making things worse by inflaming an already tense situation. Police officers generally respond best to a calm acknowledgement of wrongdoing and admission of remorse, full stop. Making up excuses, denying that you've made a mistake, challenging the police officer's knowledge of the law (even if you're right), getting angry, lippy, or hostile are all recipes for a bad interaction, and likely a bigger fine than you might otherwise have received. If your ticket was unjust, or incorrect for any reason, the place to deal with it is usually via the court system, where a rational appeal can be made and heard outside of the power-soaked setting of a street stop.

Find out what rules are in place where you live, but in some cities it is not a legal requirement to provide a piece of identification if you are pulled over on a bike. Often enough, it is acceptable to simply identify yourself and provide any additional information requested by police regarding address details. Further, in most provinces and states, your driver's licence has nothing to do with a bike riding infraction. No demerit points should be involved in a ticket.

IN CASE OF
COLLISION OR CRASH

More collisions seem to happen during the week, in warmer months, during dry conditions, and, unsurprisingly, during the morning and evening rush-hour commute on major and minor arterial roads. Spring is also a higher risk time, as many riders need a bit of time to get their "bike legs" back and reacclimatize to the roadway, and drivers need time to get used to increased bike traffic. Daylight-savings-time change in the fall often corresponds with an increased number of collisions.

However, the most common cause of injury while riding a bike is not a collision with a motor vehicle but a crash due to losing control of the bike because of some distraction or external cause (e.g., a pothole). These kinds of obstacles are usually easy enough to avoid if you stay vigilant.

What to Do When a
Collision or Crash Occurs

As much as we do our best to avoid them, collisions with motor vehicles do occasionally happen. Many people ride their entire lives with no collisions, but we all certainly experience near misses.

Here's the thing about falling down or off your bike — it's embarrassing and our first instinct is usually just to get up and get out of there. Rather than give in to the flight response, you'll want to follow along with some or all of these steps. If you're unable to do any of these things yourself, don't hesitate to ask for help from passersby.

◊ Assess yourself: Can you safely get up and get yourself and your bike out of the roadway? Do so if you're able.

◊ Call 911 to report the incident. Make sure police attend.

◊ Write down the motor vehicle's make, model, and licence plate number, and/or take a photo of it.

◊ Write down the incident report number and the investigating officer's name and badge number.

◊ Exchange contact and insurance information with the driver and witnesses, and try to record their key statements as soon as possible. Your phone likely has a way to record audio, which might be easier than writing things down. Drivers may not want to comply with this request, but you should insist.

◊ Always accept medical attention if you're in a position to do so financially. Adrenaline is powerful, and you may have an injury you are not yet aware of. This is especially important if you've hit your head or face or if your neck or back have been bent or turned.

◊ Take a few minutes to sit, calm down, call a friend, and find a nearby coffee shop, bench, or front porch to wait for pick up if needed, or just to recover yourself.

◊ Check your bike. There may be damage to your bike that is significant enough that you shouldn't ride it before it is repaired.

◊ Once you're home, be sure to take care of yourself and to document everything that you remember about the incident, any injuries you've sustained, and any damage done to your bicycle and other property (sunglasses, laptop, phone, etc.). This information is important for any future insurance claims.

◊ If you hit your head and were wearing a helmet, you'll want to assess whether a new helmet is in order. Check in with a local bike shop if you're unsure.

Keep receipts for anything related to your recovery, whether it's to do with your health or your bike and equipment. File any health or property insurance reports or claims promptly, and follow up as needed with police. In some cases, you can seek legal support if you need advice on how to proceed; there are personal injury firms that specialize in this type of incident that can give you guidance and will often provide a free consultation.

Unfortunately, there is still a widely held belief amongst police, and many drivers, that the bike rider must have done something to cause the collision. A driver who has made an error will also be defensive ("She came out of nowhere!" or "I didn't see him" are common refrains) and often try to diminish the appearance of wrongdoing, shifting the blame when telling their side. Stay calm and make sure that your version is properly understood and documented. Assert your rights as needed while maintaining deference to the attending officer.

Many of these steps apply if there was no vehicle involved. Even if you've crashed your bike, be sure to take care of yourself first and accept help if needed. Keep in mind that although collisions and falls may happen no matter how you're getting around the city, chances are you'll arrive at your destination safely.

SHARING THE ROAD AS A DRIVER

If you've got your licence, some days you may find yourself on four wheels instead of two, and there are some important things to keep in mind that can help keep roadways cooperative, rather than competitive, spaces.

» Please be patient with cyclists. They may occasionally cause you a delay, but it will be mere seconds and is not worth getting upset about. The long line of cars in front of you is usually more of a problem than a bike going around a pothole.

» Always check your blind spots for riders before making a move on city streets. It's not enough to check your mirrors — you've got to shoulder check as well.

» If the lane is too narrow to share with a bike, change lanes or slow down until there is room to pass the cyclist — it'll only take a few seconds.

» Prior to making a right-hand turn, signal and check your right-side mirrors and blind spot for cyclists to avoid cutting them off.

» Watch for oncoming riders when turning left, and remember to watch for them when looking for, and moving into, on-street parking.

» When opening your driver's-side door, use your right hand — this forces you to do a shoulder check of your blind spot.

» Communicate with cyclists through eye contact and by always using your turn signals.

» Read the road and traffic, and try to be aware of hazards nearby riders may face — do your best to anticipate their actions and give them space to manoeuvre.

» Sometimes bike riders appear to "act unpredictably," but most cyclists are just doing their best to get around weird or unsafe stuff in the road.

» Please don't use your car to intimidate someone on a bike — you may be the larger vehicle, but the bike rider has equal rights to the road.

» Passing too closely can cause you to clip a rider's handlebars. Be sure to leave at least 1 metre (3 feet) when passing, and don't follow too closely. The more space the better.

» Stopping, parking, or driving in bike lanes is illegal and puts cyclists at risk. Don't do it, even if it's "just for a minute."

» Honking is perceived as aggressive by most people. Avoid honking at cyclists, who have a right to be on the road.

» Road rage can explode out of seemingly nowhere. Do your best to keep your cool if you find yourself getting angry with a rider. If you find yourself on the receiving end of a cyclist's road rage, it's likely you've done something, consciously or not, to scare or hurt them. Try not to return the anger — listen to what they are saying because they likely would not bother engaging you if there was no reason for it. Apologize if you are able, say nothing if you're not, and give them the space to move along before driving off.

Remember that cyclists, like rivers, tend to take the path of least resistance — this occasionally means breaking a traffic rule here and there along the way. Although according to traffic laws, riders are not supposed to do these things, the "law of preservation of momentum" quite often supersedes other laws, even for drivers (ahem, rolling stops). With this in mind, try to anticipate these habits, as you do for fellow motorists, and drive accordingly.

4

Basic Maintenance

Every vehicle needs to be maintained, and bicycles are no exception. What many people forget is that riders need some upkeep too. This section will take you through the basic bike maintenance that you should at least understand, what tools are worth having in your bike kit, and also provide you with tips on keeping you and your bike in good working order.

If you live in a colder climate, are not planning to ride through the winter, and want to be ready to roll at the first signs of spring, do yourself, and your favourite bike shop or mechanic a favour, and bring your bike into the shop in the fall, when it's less busy, for a tune-up.

MAINTAINING YOUR RIDE: A STATE OF GOOD REPAIR

While I'm more of a "take it in to the bike shop" kind of person when it comes to repairs, maintenance, and installing add-ons, there are still some basic things that I know to listen and watch out for. Because my main ride, a robust and trusty Dutch city bike, has internal parts that not every bike shop mechanic has the expertise to handle, I always take it to the mechanic at the shop where I bought it. I've developed a nice relationship with the staff and owners of the shop over the years, and a visit is always a good way to catch up on local bike news. There are, however, a few basic bits of bike maintenance, and some minor repairs, that even the most mechanically challenged can take care of.

But what is involved in a tune-up? According to Reba Plummer, a worker/owner at Urbane Cyclists Co-op in Toronto, "Tune-up is a generic term that can mean anything from a minor safety check to a major overhaul ($25–$250), but every bike needs a tune-up at least once a year. A basic tune-up includes pumping up the tires, lubing the chain, adjusting the brakes and gears, and doing a bolt and bearing check. An assessment of the bike should be completed before the tune-up starts so any additional repairs (wheel truing, cable changes) or replacement parts (tire, brake pads) are included. It's always up to the rider to be aware of how their bike is functioning and ask questions of the mechanic before the work is started."

If you're comfortable getting your hands dirty and want to get to know how it all works, anyone can learn to maintain, and even repair, a basic bike, and there are great online tutorials like BicycleTutor.com that can help you. Most issues will be easy to identify if you're paying attention. While riding, listen to your bike and investigate unusual sounds, rubbing, or clicking. You may want to do the "drop test" and listen for tinkling or rattling: Hold your bike above the ground and bounce or drop it down onto the wheels. If you can identify the source, you may be able fix the problem yourself, or ask the experts.

As you ride more and get more into your bike, you'll gradually grow your set of bike tools. In the meantime, for those like myself who prefer to leave the maintenance and repairs to the experts, there are still a few things to have on hand for the most basic DIY stuff. The two absolute must-haves, for convenience and efficient riding, are a pump and chain lube. The rest are all nice-to-haves, so you can live without them.

◊ Hand pump for long rides and/or a full-sized floor pump for at home ($15–$80). It's worth

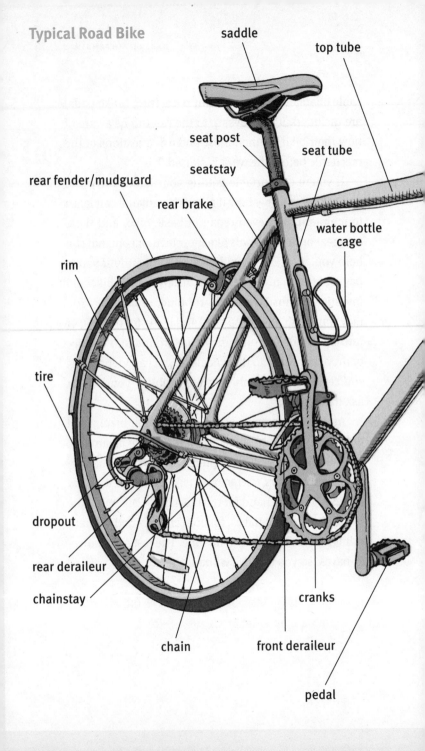

Typical Road Bike

saddle

top tube

seat post

seat tube

rear fender/mudguard

seatstay

rear brake

water bottle cage

rim

tire

dropout

rear derailleur

chainstay

chain

front derailleur

cranks

pedal

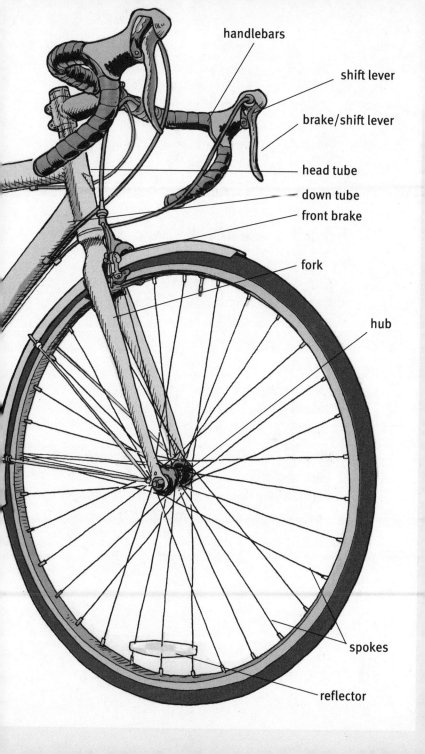

handlebars

shift lever

brake/shift lever

head tube

down tube

front brake

fork

hub

spokes

reflector

investing in a good-quality floor pump, with a head that can be used on both types of valves (description coming up) and that is robust enough to last you for years.

◊ Tire levers (usually in a set of three) for getting your bike tire on or off the wheel ($3–$6).

◊ One or two spare inner tubes ($3.50–$6).

◊ Tube patch kit ($3–$5), or you can buy a full bike repair kit with tools, tubes, patches, and the bag to hold it all in for $20–$30. (While a patch kit can be handy in a pinch, it's best to use a new tube after a flat if budget is not an issue.)

◊ A bike-specific multi-tool set, which will come in handy for adjusting handlebars and shifting or tightening your seat ($30).

◊ Bike bucket and cleaning supplies: rags, scrub brush, toothbrush, sponge, degreaser, and liquid soap (all liquids should ideally be non-toxic and hand, planet, and sewer friendly).

◊ Chain lube.

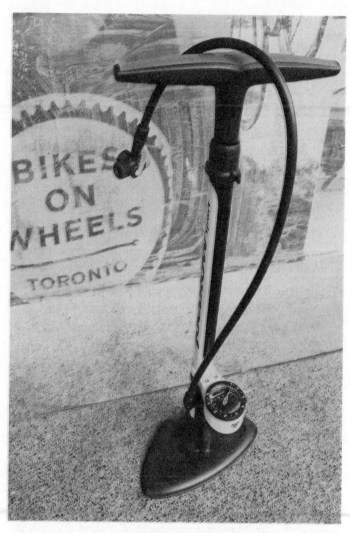

Always good to have a bike pump handy

Checking and Maintaining Tire Pressure

It's usually recommended that you check your tire pressure regularly and re-inflate as needed for optimum bike performance. Ideally you'll want to do a pressure check about once a week. I have to admit that I only started to do this consistently a couple of years ago. There'd been a number of times when I would ride around for a few days wondering why I seemed to be going slower and working harder before I clued in to the fact that my tires needed air. Sad but true — and surprisingly common. Not only does your bike not roll as fast or smoothly with low tire pressure, your tires and inner tubes are more prone to punctures. Be sure not to overinflate, or you could find yourself startled by a tube explosion and end up fixing a flat.

Although I usually just do the "thumb test," by pressing down on the tires to see if they're getting soft, the best way to check your tire pressure is with a proper floor (bike) pump — the kind that stands up on its own and has a pressure gauge. Tire manufacturers print the recommended pressure onto the side of bike tires; you want to stay within the recommended range. Road bike tires are generally higher pressure than mountain bike tires, and hybrids and city bikes will fall somewhere in between. To figure out the best tire pressure for you and your bike, visit your local bike shop and ask for their advice — jot it down for future reference. Keep in mind that air pressure in your tires goes down as the temperature drops, so add some air to your tires when the weather shifts.

There are two different types of valves on inner tubes, Shraeder and Presto. A good floor pump will have a head fitted for each so you can use the side of the head suited to the valves on your bike.

Cleaning Your Bike

In addition to your bike looking good, the ever-crucial moving parts will work better if you keep your bike clean and grime free. A full body wash and detailing should ideally be done at least once a year, but your chain and gears will need more regular attention. If they start looking dry or rusty, or make noises, they might need some TLC. The stuff you keep in your bike bucket will be just what you need.

If you've been riding through a cold winter, spring is a great time to give your bike a good wash. Road salt, grime, and grit are terrible for your chain, and all parts of your bike really, regardless of the season. Setting aside some time on the weekend once or twice a year to treat your ride to a little scrub will get the bike back into top shape and help all of its parts last longer.

If you don't have a garage or driveway in which to

wash your ride, a local coin-operated DIY car wash is the perfect place for this — grab your bike bucket and remember to bring the right coins to operate the water hose.

It's best to start by lightly hosing down your bike to remove all of the loose debris, but don't use high-pressure water on your bike: It can force water and debris into places they don't belong. Next, move on to the greasy, gritty drive chain area. Apply the degreaser and let it sit for a minute. Use a combination of rags and scrub brushes to get all of the built-up crud out of your chain links, derailleur, gears, etc. Reapply degreaser to tough spots. Once that's done, start from the top and sponge down the frame, wheels, and spokes with soapy water. Old socks make great bike-washing gloves. You can use a (non-greasy) scrub brush for the really grungy bits, like rims. Rinse thoroughly.

Chain Maintenance

Fear not, you don't have to take the chain off your bike in order to clean or lube it. You also don't always have to degrease it and scrub it 'til it shines — a monthly wipe-down with a rag to get the dirt and chunks off, followed by some lube, can work quite well for most riders.

A bike stand (if you have access to one) is extra

handy for this purpose, but you can also use the kick-stand or flip your bike upside down so that the seat and handlebars are resting on the ground. If you flip, make sure to cover your saddle with a spare rag to catch any messy drips of lube or degreaser gunk.

For a simple wipe-down, hold the rag somewhat firmly around the chain in the open area in the middle, and crank the pedals backward to run the chain through it several times to remove dirt and debris. If anything's stuck, get in there with an old toothbrush.

To apply some lube, start slowly cycling the chain backward with one hand, and then drip the lube onto the chain where it meets the chainrings. Let it sit for a minute, then give all the lubed parts a quick little wipe to remove any excess and drips. Be sure to use another rag, or at least the clean part of the one you've got — you don't want to mix dirt back in there.

Some websites suggest using WD-40 on your chain, gears, and drive chain, but citrus-based degreasers are more environmentally friendly and less harsh on your bike, and bike-specific lube, such as the Finish Line, is also preferable.

You also want to keep an eye on your chain to see if it's saggy or skipping. As with other repairs, you can do it yourself if you're confident and have the right tools, or take it in to your local shop for replacement.

Brakes

Your brakes are a key part of how you stay safe while maintaining control over your bike, so keep a regular eye on them. There are three main types of brakes: rim, disk, and drum, all of which are controlled by the brake handles mounted to your handlebars. The one exception to hand-controlled brakes is the "coaster" or "back pedal" foot brake, which functions by pushing the pedals backward.

Rim brakes, the most commonly used, are located on both the front and rear wheel, and they have rubber brake pads that squeeze both sides of the metal rim of the bike wheel to slow and stop the bike's forward motion. Rubber brake pads wear down over time and can get shifted off the rim, both of which can cause them to become less effective, as can wet cycling conditions or a wheel that is bent. Brake cables, which connect the brake handles to the brake, can also get loose or seized.

Drum, or internal, brakes are contained within an enclosed drum at the central hub of the wheel. Though they can overheat with extended continuous use, they are less subject to damage over time from weather and road debris and are a good option for year-round city riding.

Disk brakes, common on mountain bikes because of issues with rim brakes and off-road mud and debris, are also located at the hub, usually on the left side, of the front and rear wheel.

If your brakes feel funny when you squeeze the brake handles, don't slow you down fast enough, or make strange screeching sounds, it's time to take a closer look and do repairs as needed. It is not safe to ride without brakes in good working order — no brakes means no control.

Remember your ABCs:

Air pressure in your tires

Brakes that are working properly

Chain that is clean, lubed, and running well

Changing a Flat Tire

This is a pretty essential skill for anyone riding a bike and also fairly simple once you get the hang of it. That said, it's more complicated to do on, say, the rear wheel of a city bike with internal brakes and gears, so, again, I tend to leave it to the experts at my bike shop. When you get a flat, however, wheel your bike beside you, don't ride, to avoid damaging the tire or wheel rims.

While the part where you physically loosen the tire from the wheel and replace the inner tube is pretty much the same for a standard front or rear wheel, the

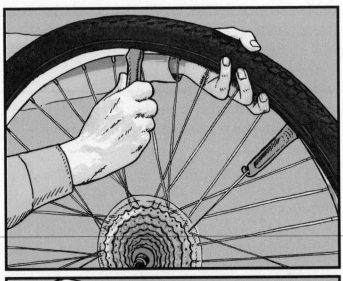

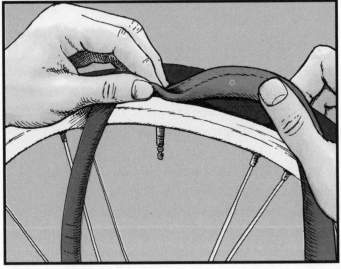

rear wheel also needs to have the chain removed and re-turned to the cogs, which can be a bit more messy. Here are the basic steps for fixing a flat, but I also recommend watching one of the many videos online and practising at home before you get stuck with a flat out on the road.

1. Release the front brakes and take the wheel off your bike using the quick-release bolts if you have them or the wrench on your multi-tool for regular bolts.

2. Take off the cap on the valve, release any re-maining air, and then unstick the tire from the rim by pushing in along the edge of the tire all along one side and then the other.

3. Wedge two of your tire levers under the edge of the tire and slide the third along to lift the tire off the rim and remove the tube.

4. Check the inside of the tire for damage or debris poking through — this is what may have caused the flat, and it needs to be removed. Your old tube may only have a small hole that could be patched (using a tube patch kit), so hang onto it and take a closer look when you've got time.

5. Pull out your new tube and use your pump to inflate it about halfway.

6. Refit one side of the tire into the wheel rim. Place the tube's valve through the hole in the rim, and feed the tube into place under the tire while trying not to twist it.

7. Push the other side of the tire back into the rim of the wheel, but avoid pinching the new tube in the process. (A pinched tube means another flat coming your way!)

8. Inflate your new tube about halfway, then check to see that everything is sitting right on the rim of the wheel.

9. Pump your tire to your regular pressure, reinstall the wheel on your bike, reconnect your brake, and be sure to check that everything is secure.

MAINTAINING YOUR BODY/ENGINE

When you're zipping around the city from one appointment to the next, it's easy to forget about your body's needs — until the next day, when your sore glutes or neck might remind you. You can't have a happy cyclist with an aching, tired body, so I've compiled a few basic tips to keep you running as smoothly as your ride.

Hydrate

Your breakfast, lunch, and dinner are the only gas your bike needs to get you around town, and staying well hydrated is equally important for us water-based creatures. Water is to your body and joints what lube is to your bike chain. Make sure you drink enough H_2O (or sports drinks, if that's your thing) before and after your ride, as well as during your ride if it's a particularly long one.

Mind Your Form

I've been stressing how important it is to stay aware of what's happening around your bike, but it's also important to pay attention to what's happening on it. Keep these things in mind, and you'll ride more comfortably and more effectively.

◊ Make sure your bike is fit properly to your body (see pages 14–16).

◊ Engage your core. It's fairly easy to forget about your abdominal muscles when regularly riding, but they give you balance and help prevent injury and strain to your back. It's always a good idea to try to fit in some core strengthening whenever you can. Try holding a plank position (resting on your elbows and your toes, with your body in a straight line) and trying variations based on your ability and comfort level.

◊ Maintain good posture. Keep in mind what your grandmother used to say: "Sit up straight, dear!" Do your back a favour and try not to slouch while riding, regardless of the type of bike you're riding.

◊ Give your neck, back, and shoulders a break. Add a basket or panniers, or both, to your bike.

◊ Adopt shock-absorber habits. Make like a mountain biker and lift yourself off your seat when you encounter a bump, pothole, or rough road. The natural bend of your knees and elbows will absorb some of the force.

◊ Know your gears. The key to efficient riding is all in the gears. You'll save yourself the irreparable wear and tear on your knees that can come from habitually straining to start up again on a green, or to ride up a hill, in the wrong gear. As Sarah B. Hood writes in her book *Practical Pedalling*, "Basically, you should always ride in the lowest gear you can."

◊ Rest the balls of your feet, not your arches, on the pedals. Human arches aren't designed for that kind of pressure, which can cause damage over time.

As with anything physical, if it hurts you might be doing it wrong. Unless you're riding in the Tour de France, or some local long-distance fundraising ride with big hills to climb, cycling should be comfortable. Anything that causes you pain in the rear, arms, neck, back, feet, or knees should be investigated and adjusted so you resolve the issue.

Stretch

Even though it's hard to make the time, ideally we would all make five minutes of stretching as much of a habit as locking our bike — especially after longer or more challenging rides. Fitness instructor Miriam Schacter notes, "Our muscles contract intensely while pumping pedals and supporting our body's frame in motion, so it makes sense to refresh and restore our muscle fibers and fascia [connective tissues like tendons and ligaments] through stretch work. We can also move lactic acid out of our systems faster with deep static stretches and breath work."

If you can take the time to do a few simple stretches after longer rides, your body will thank you. These are all stretches you can do standing by your bike when you've arrived at your destination. According to the National Academy of Sports Medicine, you'll get the most benefits if you hold each stretch for about 30 seconds a side.

◊ Quadriceps stretch: Standing on one leg, bring your other heel to your butt, keeping your knees together and your back straight. Gently engage your lower abs and think about your knee extending toward the ground. You'll feel a stretch along the front of your leg. Use a building for support or go hands-free and work on your balance. Repeat with the opposite leg.

◊ Hamstring stretch: Cross one foot in front of the other and then bend and try to touch the ground in front of you. Keep your knees soft so that the stretch you feel is in the back of your leg but not behind your knee. Relax your neck and gently shake it yes or no to release it. Roll up slowly, one vertebra at a time. Repeat with the other leg in front.

◊ Calf stretch: Start with your hands against a wall in front of you and one foot extended behind you. Keep your back knee and foot pointed forward, heel on the ground, then gently bend your front knee, lunging forward toward the

wall until you feel a stretch in the back of your
extended calf.

◊ Shoulder and wrist rotation: Roll your shoulders
up toward your ears a few times, and try pulling
back your elbows like you are kayaking. Rotate
your hands at the wrists and stretch out your
fingers.

If you want to take your stretching to the next level,
find a yoga studio you like and, with mindful practice,
your cycling, and your flexibility, should improve. Both
activities also let you practise being present. "It takes
practise to cultivate presence of mind," says Kelli Refer, author of *Pedal, Stretch, Breathe* and development
assistant at Bike Works. "Our minds tend to fixate on
the past, like when that jerk honked at you, or pon-
der the future, like wondering what is over the next
hill. When we are aware of our body, our breath, and
our surroundings we enhance our ability to adapt to
the changing circumstances of the road. When we are
aware and alert we are safer — both on our bikes and
on our yoga mats. In either activity, if you notice your
mind starting to wander, it helps to bring your focus to
your breath. Your breath is always present."

5

Cycling for All Ages

One of the best things about bicycles is that they are accessible to just about everyone — the joys of riding a bike around town are not reserved for the young and able bodied, or even for humans. This chapter explores a few adaptations that can get just about anyone out on a bicycle.

RIDING WITH KIDS

My earliest cycling memory is of sitting in my bucket seat behind my dad on his bicycle as we rode through the ravine near our condo. My parents had matching road bikes, and there was never a doubt that I'd be going along for the ride. Kids of all ages can share the joyful and practical aspects of riding, either on your bike, via an extension to it, in a cargo bike, or on their own two wheels. Bikes and families go together like toast and jam.

Although most children tend to learn to ride a bicycle on their own between five and seven years of age, as young as two or three they can start with a scoot-type push-bike that has no pedals and helps teach balance.

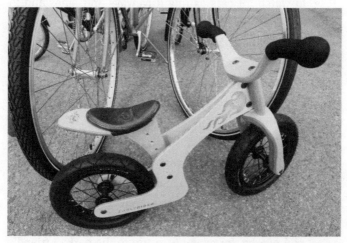

A great way for children to learn
to balance on two wheels

From what I've heard, the joy of seeing your child ride on their own bike for the first time is comparable to their thrill of accomplishment. Starting your child on a bike early will help them form healthy lifelong habits and is an excellent way to help them gain independence and confidence, as well as improve dexterity, fitness, and balance. Though the streets can seem even more threatening when your children are on two wheels, Toronto writer and cycling advocate Steve Brearton notes, "Be cautious of obvious hazards, but don't protect children from the freedom and health benefits they quickly experience. Remind them to watch for cars exiting driveways and lanes and to be careful emerging into an intersection from behind a tangle of poles and newspaper boxes. As they get older, remember to ask how comfortable they feel riding and what routes to take — studies show children perceive roads with fresh eyes and have a greater sense of risk from traffic or street."

When riding with your children, start with short local trips. Lana Stewart of ModalMom.com, adds, "You definitely want to make those first learning experiences fun. Don't start with a grocery run or doctor's appointment. Keep those first destinations interesting and nearby, for example, a trip to the park, a friend's house, or favourite place to eat. Having biking associated with good experiences will set them up for a positive outlook on using a bike to get around."

Tania Lo, mother of two and co-founder of *Momentum Mag*, has great advice about bringing your kids along for the ride: "Deciding to ride with children is a new commitment, but once you get in the rhythm of pulling your bike out, putting on the helmets, packing your extra layers and snacks, it can take less time than putting the kids in a car seat and loading up the trunk. Sometimes it's even less of a hassle than getting in a car or depending on public transit."

As with everything else discussed in this book, there are vast additional resources available in print and online publications specific to cycling for and with children. With so many options for child seats, trail-a-bikes, trailers, cargo bikes, and kids bikes now available, one could write a book on just that alone. So here are some basics, safety guidelines, and rules of the road for riding with your kids.

Bike Seats and Trailers

Very young children will generally learn about cycling by being taken along for the ride. Cities permit biking with children but require young passengers and riders to wear a helmet and be properly secured in approved bike seats and trailers. Any bike seat, tag-along attachment, or carrier should work for you and your child, but before riding with your child you must be a capable and confident rider yourself. Lisa Logan, Toronto bike mom and lifelong urban cyclist, advises, "The carrier is only as safe or good as your riding skills. Statistics are meaningless if you are not riding with confidence. The parent should always choose what suits their lifestyle and comfort first. Kids are very adaptable, and while they may scream or squirm the first time on a new seat, they will most likely quickly grow to love it."

Parents with very young children have two options, bike seats and trailers.

Children's Bike Seats or Carriers ($80–$240) are small seats that mount to the bike frame. It's generally recommended to have a child's bike seat installed correctly at a trusted bike shop. Extra care should also be taken to keep the bike steady while mounting, dismounting, and riding, to properly secure the child in place, and to make sure that the child's feet, arms, and clothing don't get caught in the bike's spokes or other moving parts.

Carriers are less expensive than trailers, but they can also be, in general, more dangerous. Kids can fall out of the carrier seat if the bike tips over or if the seat is not properly secured, causing serious injury or quite a scare at the very least. Further, a one-to-two-year-old child and bike seat add extra weight to the bike and can affect your balance and stability, especially in the event of quick turns and abrupt stops. Practise riding with just the bike seat to get used to the feeling and balance of your bike with this new attachment. Add your child when you feel comfortable. The American

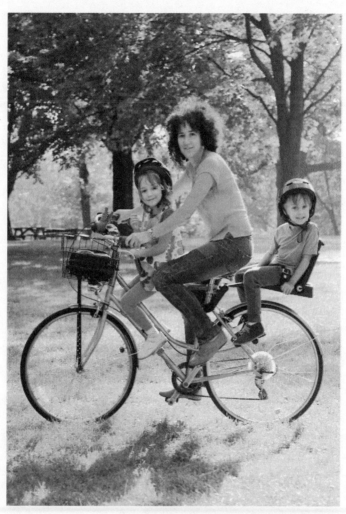

With added child seats, this becomes
a bicycle built for three

Academy of Pediatrics recommends that kids be at least one year old before riding along in a bike seat.

Bike Trailers ($200–$1,000) are generally safer for transporting kids and allow for naps, although they're usually more expensive than kids' seats. The average trailer is equipped with two wheels for stability and has waterproof and/or mesh screen covers to block sun, bad weather, and bugs. Depending on the design, trailers can be connected to the seat post or the rear wheel hub, and they are usually easy to attach and remove. You can purchase a second hitch if more than one parent will be using the trailer. The best trailers have a five-point harness, can be adapted for kids of different sizes, and have adequate covering. As always, visibility on the road is important, and since bike trailers are also lower to the ground, you'll want to attach red tail lights and reflectors for night riding and a tall, bright bike flag to make it more noticeable to motorists, pedestrians, and other cyclists during the day.

Trailer Cycles ($125–$250), also known as tag-along bikes and trail-a-bikes, are an option for older kids. These have one- or two-wheeled extensions that attach to the seat post or a specialized rack on the back of an adult-sized bike. Trailer cycles allow older kids, aged three to six, to pedal along or take a break as needed. These attachments are usually easy to take on and off and won't affect the main bike much when in action. You'll feel as though you're hauling something though, and movements your child makes from side to side can be noticeable but easily handled if you are a confident rider. These can be an excellent option for dropping off your child somewhere — the tag-along can be removed and securely locked so that you can proceed unencumbered to your destination. Lights, as always, are needed at night, and a rear light should be placed on the trailer cycle.

Various cargo bikes (see pages 32–33 for more info) can also be used to transport your children, whether it means putting them in the front box compartment of a bakfiets or on the back of a longtail addition complete with a child seat or safety hoops.

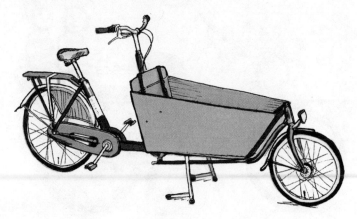

Consumer Reports has an excellent multi-page guide to buying and using carrier seats and trailers, so check it out online if you're considering these options for biking with kids.

Kids and attachments can add extra weight to bikes, sometimes up to 45 kilograms (100 pounds), so make sure that you are in good enough shape and are confident enough in your cycling skills to pull the load. If you can afford the investment, adding electric assist to your bike, or buying an electric bike, can be a great way to make hauling the extra weight of kids, cargo, and carriers more manageable.

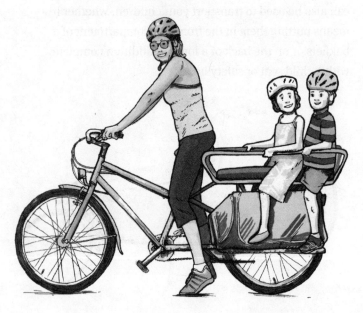

Whatever add-ons you may use, most of which can be purchased second-hand from other families whose kids have outgrown them, keep in mind kids' bikes and trailers are just as readily stolen as adult bikes, so be sure to buy an additional high-quality lock for your trailer and kids bikes and always lock them up after use, through the bike or trailer frame, even if you are storing them inside a garage. Combine a thick and extra long cable with a smaller sturdy U-lock to secure all the smaller items together, and connect them to a fence or other secure object if one is available where you're storing them.

Tips for Riding with Children

Teaching your kids to ride in an urban environment means there are a lot of rules to learn and hazards to manage. Remember, you're not just developing skills, you're developing and building awareness. Ryan J. Rusnak, city planner in Davenport, Iowa, notes, "I spend a great deal of time developing my children's cycling awareness, which really means minimizing risk. A few of our daily utterances include 'car up' — there is a car ahead, 'hold your line' — ride in a straight line, and 'clear' — there are no cars left or right and we may proceed through an intersection. What a joy to hear my child shout, 'Car back, Dad.'"

The Bike Madison website (of Madison, Wisconsin) has some helpful tips on teaching kids the ins and outs of biking in urban areas, and I've summarized them for you here.

◊ Kids should always wear a helmet, and they are required by law in every U.S. and Canadian city up to various ages.

◊ Depending on the city, kids are often permitted to ride on sidewalks up to a certain age (this varies) in order to prepare them for street cycling.

◊ Parents should teach kids about common sidewalk hazards such as pedestrians, dogs, signs, blind spots around corners and buildings, opening shop doors, and fire hydrants.

◊ Kids should also be aware of proper riding etiquette: giving pedestrians the right of way, warning others before passing with their voice or bell, slowing down as needed, and stopping at driveways and intersections.

◊ Just like adults, kids should learn to shoulder check. To help them learn this skill, ride behind them and occasionally call out their name to get them used to quickly checking over their left shoulder while continuing to ride straight.

◊ Have kids mimic hand signals at first and then use them on their own.

◊ Make sure that your kids' bikes are the right size and well maintained. A good-fitting, regularly inspected bike is a safer bike for kids to ride.

◊ Don't forget water and snacks to keep kids fuelled.

◊ Protective eyewear, sunscreen, and a hat (under a helmet) are all essential.

Riding While Pregnant

Many cyclists are comfortable continuing to ride into various stages of their pregnancy. A step-through frame can make getting on and off the bike easier, and riding can often be more comfortable than walking or taking transit. It's really about your level of comfort and perception of risk based on your riding habits. As a confident rider, you should make your own decision and ignore what busybodies have to say about your choice. This is also something worth discussing with a partner early in your pregnancy. Stop riding when you decide it's the right time for you to do so.

RIDING AS WE AGE

Perhaps your jogging habit has taken a toll on your knees, you're tired of poor public transit options, you've decided you no longer want a car, or maybe you're thinking it's time to get more active again. Low-impact cycling can help with all of those things, and moderate daily exercise remains important as we get older, in particular to help maintain functional health and to prevent loss of bone and muscle mass. If you plan to start cycling again, be sure to check in with your doctor, and pay special attention to the strategies for taking care of your body outlined in Chapter 4.

Keep in mind that reaction times and reflexes change with age, and it becomes increasingly important to go at a pace that suits your ability to safely respond to the dynamics of an active roadway and the controlled chaos of off-road paths shared with pedestrians, children, and dogs. Falls and collisions can have a more significant impact on an aging body, and our ability to heal from injury is also affected. According to an Organisation for Economic Cooperation and Development (OECD) report on cycling safety, the elderly tend to suffer "more severe consequences due to lessened overall physical condition, often more brittle bones, less elastic soft tissue, weakened locomotive functions including reaction times."

For these reasons, it's even more important to ride predictably, follow the rules of the road, find the right bike or trike for your ability level, and only ride in places where you are confident and comfortable. Remember, the overall health and social benefits of riding for transportation and recreation still far outweigh the health risks of crashes.

Bike Styles

In addition to everything listed in Chapter 1 regarding bike fit, handlebar styles and positions, and types of bicycles, there are a few additional things to keep in mind for older riders or people with mobility challenges.

◊ Do you need a bike that can accommodate specific physical limitations or that is easy to get on and off of?

◊ Will you be able to propel the bike under your own steam or would electric assistance make for a safer or more enjoyable ride?

◊ Where will you store your bike? Ideally, you should find a place to lock it up that does not require you to lift the bike off the ground or carry it for any distance. Most bikes are fairly heavy, and even riders in their teens and 20s through 40s struggle to lift and carry their bikes. You are at greater risk of injury from a fall or strain while lifting and carrying your bike as you age, so avoid it if you're able and ask for help as needed.

◊ Do you still have good balance, or would three wheels make you more comfortable and confident?

Variations on your standard bicycle can accommodate many of these concerns, and I'll go over some of the more popular choices.

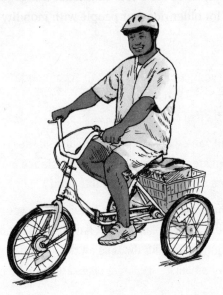

Adult Tricycles are a particularly good choice for anyone concerned about maintaining their balance while riding. Having two wheels in the back makes these extra stable, plus they have a big basket that makes them super handy for confidently running errands. I'm fairly certain there will be a pedal-assist tricycle in my golden years.

Tandem Bicycles are fantastic bikes for social rides and for riding with a friend or partner that needs assistance due to physical challenges, such as vision loss or decreased physical strength. The stronger rider takes the lead position and maintains control of the bike, while the rear rider helps add more power by pedalling when able.

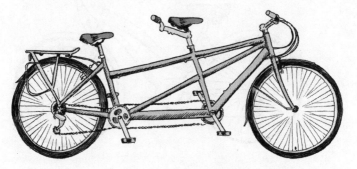

Electric Assistance packages can be useful if you have longer distances to travel, tire easily, or need a little extra help dealing with hills. The other option, if you're in the market for a new bike altogether, is to shop around for an e-bike (throttle and motor power on demand) or pedelec (power-assistance when pedalling). There are many varieties, shapes, and sizes now on the market, although some e-bikes are quite heavy so may be too cumbersome.

Comfort Bikes are designed for easygoing riding on paved surfaces and for maximum ease of use. They are a blend of hybrid and cruiser bikes and provide an upright position that also allows you to easily put your foot down without getting off your seat.

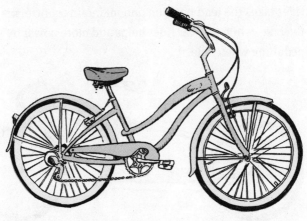

Recumbents and Semi-recumbents are another breed of bicycle altogether, offering a reclining seated position that means the rider's weight is more broadly

distributed. This extra comfort also comes with reduced balance and manoeuvrability, so be sure to do
your research and road test them well. They're also less
visible to drivers because of their low profile, so they're
not ideal for riding in city traffic.

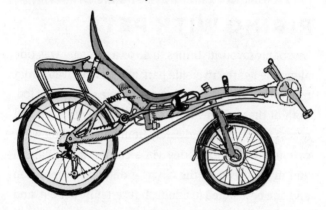

Custom-made Bicycles can be built or adapted to accommodate differently abled riders.

Depending on the number and variety of bike shops
where you live, you may or may not be able to find these
styles of bike locally. Most quality bike shops should be
able to help you identify, order, and assemble the type,
model, and fit of bike best suited to you. Shopping online is also an option, though you'll still want to ask
for help with assembly at a local bike shop to ensure
that you've got it properly put together. Additionally,

barring custom-made bikes, you should also be able to find most of these second-hand via newspaper ads, garage sales, or online. Remember to follow the tips for buying a used bike on page 18.

RIDING WITH PETS

One of my favourite things to do as a teenager was ride along the nearby riverside park bike path or waterfront trail with my dog, Trixie. I'm pretty sure she loved it too. Both of these routes were off-street paths that I could access fairly easily and safely from home. Riding with, carrying, or towing a dog via a carrier on residential and main streets of the city is a different proposition and one best suited to adults, but certainly doable, and increasingly common among more confident cyclists of any age. When I dog-sit my sister's toy poodle, Bonny, she and her blanket regularly come for a spin in the front basket of my city bike — it's a sight to behold and a convenient way to visit friends and to get her to the big off-leash dog park she prefers.

Local and online pet and bike shops are a great place to check out the various products that are available to you and your furry friend, but here are some ideas to get you started.

Pets as Passengers

Small dogs can be carried in many standard open handlebar baskets; dog-specific open, covered, or enclosed front baskets; or in certain types of rear baskets or panniers. The enclosed baskets could presumably also be used for cats, if you're brave enough to try to wrangle a cat for a bike ride.

People have been using custom-built or kid-specific trailers for this purpose for years, but there are now many open, covered, or enclosed trailer models made specifically with different-sized dogs in mind. The side bonus of owning a detachable trailer is that it can also

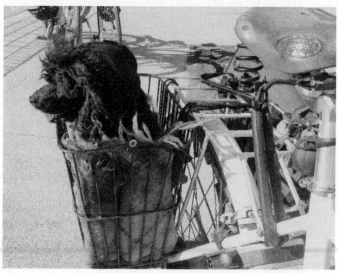

Along for the ride and loving it!

be used for things like grocery shopping. Remember to buy an additional high-quality lock for the trailer, and store it indoors if possible. Some trailers also fold for easy storage, and most enclosed trailers have good ventilation and rain protection features.

Dogs of all sizes can also join you via cargo bike and often enjoy the ride as much as the kids seem to. Some dogs will take to travel by bike naturally, while others will need to get used to the idea. Nervous dogs can do things like jump out of a moving cargo bike or basket, so try this type of carrying in a park rather than on the road when you're first introducing your pet to cycling, and make use of a safety harness if needed.

Running Dogs Alongside

If you can confidently incorporate it, riding with your dog running along beside you is one of the best ways for your dog to get a good run without exhausting yourself or requiring another dog to play with. You both win by getting out and about together for some fun, exercise, and adventure.

That said, don't let Fido come along for the ride without training. Not all dogs will be keen on running beside a bike — some are petrified of the things — so start slowly and see what works for your canine companion. You should also always keep your dog on-leash, and be extra careful with dogs prone to distraction and sudden bursts of energy. If you're planning to cycle with your dog beside you on paths, your best bet is to start getting them used to this from a relatively young age, but only once some basic training has been achieved. Always be careful with your bike around your dog — a traumatic experience early on can become an insurmountable obstacle. Start slow, even just walking your bike and dog together for a while, try some short rides, keep an eye on how they're doing, and change pace accordingly. According to the Ottawa Humane Society, there are a few commands to teach your dog that can help: "Ready," "Hike (let's go!)," "Gee (right)," "Haw (left)," "Whoa (slow down)," and "Stop." You'll sound a bit like a dogsledder, but you'll end up with a smoother, safer ride for both of you.

Biking with your dog is best suited to bike or shared off-street paths, side streets, or, if needed for a short distance, main streets with bike lanes or cycle tracks. If riding on busier streets for any distance, keep your bike between your dog and traffic whenever possible, and have them run along the edge of the sidewalk where feasible on side streets — while being mindful of pedestrians and obstacles of course. As always, if in doubt, move to the sidewalk and walk it out. When riding with your dog at night, consider adding a flashing bike light to their collar or harness and putting a reflective vest on them if any part of your ride is on street. And keep in mind that only the most experienced winter riders should attempt to bring along a dog for a run if the roads and paths are snowy or icy.

While the easiest thing to do may be to just hold your dog's leash and start riding with them right beside you, it isn't necessarily the safest option. You might let go of the leash if your dog lunges suddenly, losing control of the dog and possibly your bike. That's where the many varieties of dog-walking bike attachments come in. Some, like a tow leash, are mounted at the rear of the bike and allow you to keep your hands leash-free and your dog at a safe distance from the pedals and wheels. Some models include shock-absorbing spring coils to decrease the effect of lunges and pulling. To decrease

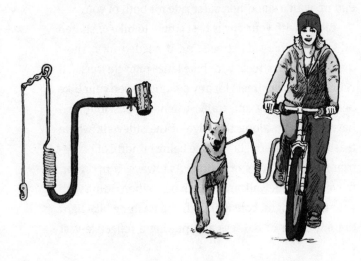

strain on your dog's neck, connecting the attachment to a properly fitted harness is preferable to a collar. It's important to remember that the surface of the road or path may be too hot or rough on your dog's paws. Our furry companions also don't know when to stop and are likely to keep running beyond the point of exhaustion. Take water breaks, keep an eye on their paws, and time your ride so that you take the run home into account. Just as with humans who are starting a regular running habit, start with shorter rides and build up your dog's endurance. Cycling with your dog(s) can be really fun and is worth trying once you're confident on your bike.

6

Advocacy and the Future of Cycling

By now you've got all of the information you need to buy, maintain, and ride your bike; you've got a good sense of the rules of the road and how to plan your route; and you've either been riding more often or are totally ready to hit the road. But is the road ready for you? Most cities in North America are making some effort to fit bikes in, but given the huge interest in cycling and the general need to move increasingly large populations of people, they're not doing it nearly fast enough. Which is why your trusty local cycling advocates and political champions are so important. Bike advocates argue for and support the inclusion of bicycles into all aspects of our transportation systems and city planning, working directly and indirectly on behalf of anyone riding a bicycle. Without their diligent and tireless efforts, our cities would be far less bikeable and quite likely more hostile to the people choosing to ride.

Many of the advocacy organizations across North America are supported through, and partially or fully funded by, members. Engaged local cyclists pay an annual membership fee to enjoy member benefits but primarily to support policies for safer riding conditions. And members get a lot for their investment! Bike advocates coordinate campaigns; work directly with politicians and bureaucrats; consult on policy development; organize special events, workshops, and training; develop educational resources; and much more. Believe me, as someone who's worked as a full-time cycling advocate, I can assure you it takes all of this and then some to shift the status quo, lock in bike-related improvements at the policy level, and see them manifested on our shared public roadways.

Since early 1901, when the American Automobile Association was formed, car advocates and lobbyists have been driving the political agenda when it comes to transportation policy and planning. It's no secret that many drivers, who still far outnumber cyclists, remain frustrated with a changing environment and unhappy about having to share the road with what some consider a child's toy and others still view as a substandard vehicle for the have-nots in society. Issues of dominance, Darwinian survival of the fittest, money, power, and entitlement are all in play on city roadways and in the hallways of political power. Every inch of cycling facilities has been won by fighting the good fight and activating the power of political will.

Political will is the fundamental difference between those cities that have adapted policies and begun to successfully and safely integrate bicycles and those that have not. Given how little actual money is required, compared to similar public transit and highway projects, where there's a political will, there's always a way. Political champions know how to tap into and build public and political support for projects that matter, and bike advocates know how to find, nurture, and support political champions.

Many smart and forward-thinking municipal governments in North America have begun to see the light (and return on investment) when it comes to bicycles and bike infrastructure, welcoming it as a very real part of the solution for moving people more efficiently while also improving the quality of life of their citizens. Take New York City for example: The recent bicycle renaissance, thanks in large part to the installation of over 320 kilometres (200 miles) of new bike lanes, cycle tracks, along with a public bike-share system in Manhattan, is remarkable. This was part of a long battle that, while facilitated by a transportation commissioner and mayor with a strong and determined vision, came following years of advocacy work on the part of organizations like Transportation Alternatives.

"Sometimes the pace of bicycle improvements might seem glacial and frustrating," says Clarence Eckerson Jr., director of Streetfilms. "But the worldwide momentum has been building and is now stronger than ever. I still recall the mid-1990s, when there were some days I wouldn't see another bike commuter (or pedestrian!) on my a.m. journeys over the Brooklyn Bridge. Today, savvy cyclists avoid the bridge when they can because it is so congested with people on foot and bikes at all times of the day. Incremental change might not be the most exciting, but over time adds up."

It was only in 1987 that New York's mayor at the time tried and almost succeeded in banning bicycle riding in the heart of Midtown Manhattan to stop bike messengers from allegedly "causing dangerous traffic chaos." It shouldn't be news to you that messengers kick traffic's ass, they don't cause it. So dramatic, timely, and well received was the change in New York's approach to public space and transportation policy that the transportation commissioner responsible for it, Janette Sadik-Khan, has become somewhat of a celebrity in urban planning circles and former New York City mayor Michael Bloomberg was appointed as the United Nations special envoy for cities and climate change.

One of the greatest misconceptions about the various types of dedicated bicycle infrastructure is that they only serve a minority of the population — that they're pet projects for bicyclists. The reality is that whether you're left or right leaning, urban or suburban, rich or poor, bikes are simply one of the most accessible and efficient forms of urban mobility. While they mean much more than that to some people, at the heart of the matter is our fundamental right to choose how we move and make our way through life. Just like sidewalks, bike lanes and cycle tracks serve all road users by providing a clearly marked space for a specific user group and, in turn, adding to the safety and predictability of the roadway. That safety and predictability, in particular when reliably networked, means more riders from all walks of life.

Not only do bike facilities make visible the fact that cycling is a viable way to move around the city and demonstrate the commitment on the part of municipal governments to encourage travel by bike, these facilities help many who might otherwise be too nervous to ride add two-wheeled travel to their transportation options. In fact, their addition to urban roadways — networked and physically separated cycle tracks in particular — is the single most important factor in the growth of ridership. According to the first multi-city academic study of U.S. protected bike lanes (2014),

"When protected bike lanes are added to a street, bike traffic rises — by an average of 75 percent in their first year alone, for the eight projects studied."

And building this type of infrastructure to accommodate bike traffic is cheap too. "One thing I like to remind my business-minded friends and colleagues about," says April Economides, president of Green Octopus Consulting, "is that bicycling is more taxpayer-friendly than driving. Bicycle infrastructure is considerably cheaper to construct than car infrastructure, the most famous example being that Portland, Oregon's outstanding 300-mile [482 km] bike network completed through year 2008 cost the same amount as one mile [1.6 km] of freeway."

But we still have a long way to go to meaningfully integrate bicycles into our urban planning and traffic systems, build real public support and understanding regarding their value, and grow the percentage of the population using bikes for transportation. As per a 2013 OECD study on cycling safety, "The traffic system does not typically account for the specific characteristics of cyclists and bicycles. . . . Though cycling is an important component of urban mobility, cyclists are often seen as intruders in the road system."

Intruders, eh? The days when the bicycle was the only vehicle (other than horse drawn carriages) on the road seem to be long forgotten. But rest assured, bikes are too important a part of the solution to urban congestion to be ignored. People need to move and bikes get the job done.

Copenhagen, the often-mentioned example of a cycling mecca of sorts, was once as car obsessed and addled as any North American city. The reason they're now so well adapted to cycling, and able to boast about having nearly 40 per cent of their population commuting by bike, is because of the citizen activism, political will, and foresight to make substantial and separated bicycle facilities a priority. Confronted with the realities of the oil crisis in the early 1970s, making non oil-dependent bicycle transportation feasible for their citizens became part of Copenhagen's city-building mandate. Consistent commitment on the part of government was the key to this success.

Mikael Colville-Andersen, Urban Mobility Expert and CEO of Copenhagenize Design Co., has noticed other cities making big changes: "It's not about Copenhagen and Amsterdam anymore; it's about the cities who have done amazing things in only six or seven years. There were no bicycles left, just a few years ago, in cities like Seville, Barcelona, Paris, Bordeaux, Dublin, or Buenos Aires. Now these cities are well on their way to reestablishing the bicycle as transport. The common denominators? Bike share systems that kick-start the return of the bicycle. Infrastructure that gives people space to ride the bikes, keeps them safe, and makes them feel safe. Traffic calming that slows down the cars, prioritizes cycling and walking. Buenos Aires has put in 140 kilometres [86 miles] of protected cycle tracks in just two years. Eighty per cent of the roads in Barcelona are now 30 km/h [18 mph] zones. Seville went from 0.2 per cent on bicycles to 7 per cent in just five years thanks to cycle tracks. Potential bicycle users need infrastructure and encouragement. It's that simple."

North American cities don't need to morph into European cities: There are ways to apply and adapt some of the best practices from successful bike cities. The most important consideration is that "traffic" includes all vehicles, and bicycles are vehicles. Bicycles, just like cars, must be incorporated into all aspects of our city-building dialogue — progressive urban planning that facilitates and encourages walking and cycling as active transportation is vital to the future of our cities and the key to our collective health.

So, what can you do? Let's say for example that you're interested in riding with your children to school or having them ride there themselves. What types of changes on the streets in your community and/or on the school grounds would make it safer for them to do so? Is there adequate bike parking? Are there bike lanes leading toward the school? Do parents in cars leave enough room for kids arriving by bike? What are the speed limits in the school zone and are people following them? Does the school ever organize Bike Rodeos to help teach the children bike skills? You can become a local bike advocate by looking into these things and working with other interested parents, teachers, school administrators, and your local bike advocacy organization to implement changes that will improve safety and help encourage more parents and kids to ride to school.

It's possible says Cycle Toronto's executive director, Jared Kolb: "We can create safer streets for cyclists, but we must communicate that need to our elected officials. Change is possible, but not without the active engagement of local communities."

Further, does your local school incorporate cycling education? By teaching children road safety, and training them to safely ride bicycles on roadways as part of the curriculum, they gain an early sense of independence and confidence, become better prepared for driving, and, in the long term, we'll have a cycling population that is more aware of road rules and on-street etiquette. In the meantime, there's a need for broad public education that can speak to all road users and make clear the roles, rights, and responsibilities of every mode of travel, along with examples of how our behaviour and misbehaviour impact all those road users around us. And if you don't want to take on your own

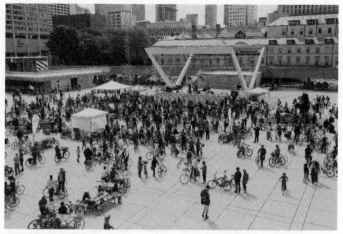

Advocacy in action — cyclists attend Bikestock
outside Toronto City Hall

campaign, check out what your local advocacy group is
up to. Maybe now is a good time to buy a membership,
attend events, or even consider volunteering some
of your time to help improve your city while learning
more about riding in it.

Getting involved can be tremendously rewarding
and motivational, says Nancy Smith Lea, director of
the Toronto Centre for Active Transportation, who took
the fight for cycling rights to the next level: "I remember the first time I rode a bike in the city. It was scary
and liberating, both at the same time. When I was hit
by a car as a new cyclist, I considered not riding my
bike anymore. Instead, I took a cycle training course to

tackle my fears and began advocating for a bike lane on the street where I was hit. Now, whenever I ride on that fantastic bike lane, I'm so glad I stuck with it."

While advocacy is quite focused on improving the on-street conditions for riders, advocates also spend a fair bit of time trying to encourage more people to take up cycling as a form of transportation. And as we've discussed, it's working. There are more people riding than ever before across North America. The more riders on city streets, the safer those streets generally become — more cyclists increase the visibility of bikes amongst the rest of traffic, and drivers become more aware of the need to share the road. That said, the only way to systematically and fundamentally reduce risk is to enhance on-street bike facilities while also educating both drivers and cyclists about how to safely use these facilities and share the roadway.

And we all, regardless of mode of travel, have so much to gain from having more people safely riding on our city streets. More people riding means fewer people sitting alone in cars in block after block of bumper-to-bumper traffic. More people riding acts as a pressure release valve for aging and overcrowded public transportation systems. More people riding means a healthier, happier population and decreased medical costs. More people riding means improvements to air quality and a reduction in noise pollution. More people riding means more money for the local economy and higher property values.

San Francisco–based advocate Chris Carlsson notes, "Bicycles in streets make them safer for everyone, and reanimate avenues as public spaces full of conversations and serendipitous connections. The bicycle is not just practical though. It is also a device that opens a door to new ways of thinking, new ways of imagining how we can make daily life together. Riding together we can make the path to a world of our own (re)design."

If all of this seems overwhelming or far-fetched, remember that just riding your bicycle safely and responsibly is an act of advocacy. If you've decided to make the switch, know that there will be moments of resistance — you'll come up with any number of reasons why driving or taking public transit today is the right thing to do. Sometimes it may be. But far more often than not, if you can work past the resistance, you'll be glad you did.

By reading this book and applying the lessons learned, you'll be well on your way to a healthy and fulfilling relationship with urban cycling. Riding a bike is to most, even those who've been at it for a long time, a daily act of courage. It's also one that has handsome rewards. Even if it's just one day a week, the best time to get started is now. Enjoy the ride!

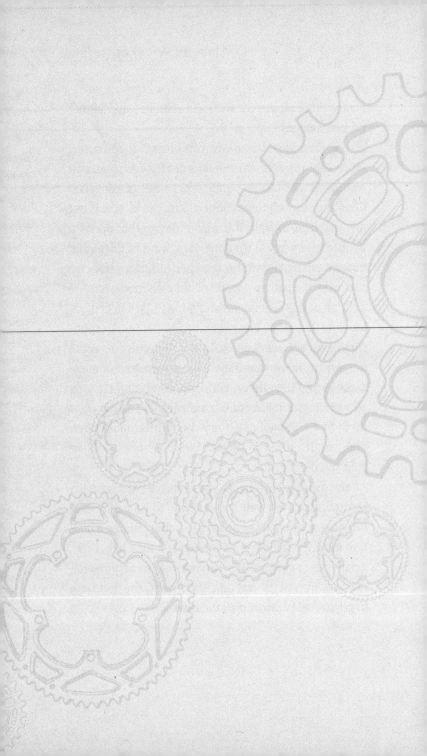

Resource Guide

Though individual cities may have specific cycling organizations, the following organizations and publications are a great start for more urban cycling intel.

GENERAL

Association of Bicycle and Pedestrian Professionals (apbp.org) Network of sustainable transportation experts.

Bicycle Benefits (bicyclebenefits.org) Reward program that offers discounts for biking in the U.S.

Bike Collectives Network (bikecollectives.org) Hub for those involved in non-profit bike collectives. The wiki offers a great list of community bike organizations around the world.

Bike Hacks (bikehacks.com) All kinds of cool, interesting, and useful stuff for your bike, from the funky to the functional. Great DIY tips.

BikeyFace (bikeyface.com) Fun web comic focused on cycling lifestyle that also raises awareness and advocates for safer streets for all.

Bike Share (bikeshare.com/map/) List of links to all the bike share programs running, or making pre-launch preparations, in cities across North America.

Canadian Cyclist (canadiancyclist.com) News site covering all aspects of cycling in Canada.

Cargo Bikes in Canada (cargobike.ca) Guide to cargo bike retailers in Canada.

City Bike Reddit (search "City name + Bicycling or Cycling + Reddit") Social news and entertainment website with sub-threads for nearly every North American city packed with all kinds of information on absolutely everything related to cycling.

Cycle Canada (cyclecanada.com) National cycling organization promoting all things bike related in Canada.

Cycle Love (cyclelove.net/archive) Photo-heavy London, England, based blog and culture site about cycling.

Disabled Sports USA (disabledsportsusa.org/cycling) Organization that provides sports and recreation opportunities to youth and adults with disabilities.

Girl Bike Love (girlbikelove.com) Group and website

with a mandate of empowering more women to take on two wheels, whether for recreational riding, commuting, or racing.

Lovely Bicycle (lovelybike.blogspot.ca) A wide-ranging blog by a beginner turned obsessive cyclist.

Loving the Bike (lovingthebike.com) Online cycling magazine with regular blog entries.

Momentum Magazine (momentummag.com) Independent print and online magazine with a focus on urban cycling. Distributed across Canada and the U.S.

A New Bike (anewbike.com) Cycling stories and culture site with lots of great photographs.

Pedestrian and Bicycle Information Center (pedbike info.org) Organization that promotes safe walking and cycling.

Sheldon Brown (sheldonbrown.com/glossary) A glossary of bike-related posts from the online guru for DIY bike repair.

Streetfilms (streetfilms.org) Streetfilms produces educational films about sustainable transportation with the goal of inspiring people worldwide.

Totcycle (totcycle.com) Seattle-based blog and culture site about bicycling with kids.

The Urban Country (theurbancountry.com) A blog all about urban cycling that has lots of cool images.

Urban Velo (urbanvelo.org) Print and online magazine that covers all things urban cycling.

Velo Joy (velojoy.com) Cycling resource and culture site primarily geared toward female cyclists.

ADVOCACY

Active Transportation (activetransportation.ca) Canadian organization advocating sustainable transport in Canada, with emphasis on bicycling.

Alliance for Biking and Walking (bikewalkalliance.org) Organization that creates and brings together and supports state/province and local bicycle and pedestrian advocacy organizations.

America Bikes (americabikes.org) Non-profit organization that advocates in Congress for bike and pedestrian initiatives.

Bicycle Law (bicyclelaw.com) Bob Mionske is a lawyer and former Olympic and pro cyclist who offers advice for cyclists who have been injured by motorists, unsafe road conditions, or defective cycling products. Contains links to Bob's publications on bicycle law and cyclists' rights.

Canada Bikes (canadabikes.org) Non-profit organization working to increase cycling in Canada.

International Bicycle Fund (ibike.org) Non-governmental, non-profit advocacy organization with global projects that focus on bike safety, education, urban planning and responsible bike tourism.

League of American Bicyclists (bikeleague.org) This organization represents bicyclists through information, advocacy, and promotion to create safer roads, stronger communities, and a bicycle-friendly America.

National Center for Bicycling and Walking (bikewalk.org) Program by the Project for Public Spaces that aims to create bike- and pedestrian-friendly American cities.

Otesha Project (otesha.ca) Sustainability focused national youth-led charitable organization that engages and inspires Canadians with hands-on learning, theatre and bicycle tours.

People for Bikes (peopleforbikes.org) The leading movement to improve bicycling in the U.S., it helps Americans to boost bicycling on a national level for results that can be seen locally.

Sustainable Cities Collective (sustainablecitiescollective.com) Website dedicated to rethinking urbanism. Often discusses urban cycling.

World Bicycle Relief USA (worldbicyclerelief.org) The non-profit World Bicycle Relief distributes bicycles in the developing world to facilitate access to healthcare, education, and encourage economic development.

ROUTE PLANNING & TOURING

Adventure Cycling Association (adventurecycling.org) Non-profit bicycle travel organization that offers tours, routes and maps, an online store, and how-to resources.

Bikemap (bikemap.net) Online tool that allows you to create and share bike route maps anywhere in the world.

Passion Vélo (passionvelo.ca) French-language website connecting cycling enthusiasts in Canada and around the world. Good source of information on bike routes, maps, etc.

Rails to Trails (railstotrails.org) American non-profit organization focused on transforming former rail lines into a nationwide network of trails.

Ride the City (ridethecity.org) Essential bicycle route-mapping site. Can be used to find bike routes for major cities in North America, South America, and Europe.

Senior Cycling Bike Tours (seniorcycling.com) Cycling tours specifically for active seniors.

Trans Canada Trail (tctrail.ca) One of the world's longest networks of trails that when completed will stretch nearly 24,000 kilometres across Canada, with path running between the Arctic, Atlantic, and Pacific oceans.

Velo Hospitality (velohospitality.com) Network of bike-friendly services in Canada and around the world. Search for bike shops, cycling clubs, and bike tours.

SAFETY

Bike Light Database (bikelightdatabase.com) Bike light buyer's guide with detailed product reviews.

CAA Bike Safety (bikesafety.caa.ca/cyclists) Resource for road sharing techniques for cyclists and motorists in Canada.

Consumer Reports Bike Trailer Buying Guide (con sumerreports.org/cro/bike-trailers/buying-guide.htm) Offers criteria for selecting a bike seat or trailer and information on various models.

Cycle-Helmets (cycle-helmets.com) Website with guides to bike helmet laws in Canada, the United States, England, Ireland, Australia, and New Zealand.

National Highway Traffic Safety Administration Bike Safety (nhtsa.gov/bicycles) U.S. government site that is ground zero for bike safety.

Ride Smart (bikeleague.org/ridesmart) The League of American Bicyclists' education program.

TRAINING AND CONDITIONING

Bike PT (bikept.com) Excellent online source for info about bike induced pains and strains and the biomechanics of bicycling.

Can Bike (canbikecanada.ca) Can Bike offers courses on cycling safely for children and adults.

Women's Cycling Canada (womenscycling.ca) Training resource site focusing on skills, training, and nutrition for female cyclists.

Selected References

Alter, Lloyd. "How much does it cost to commute by bike?" *TreeHugger*. May 26, 2011. http://www.treehugger.com/bikes/how-much-does-it-cost-to-commute-by-bike.html.

Boyd, H., M. Hillman, A. Nevill, Pearce, L.P., and B. Tuxworth. "Health-related Effects of Regular Cycling on a Sample of Previous Non-exercisers, Resume of Main Findings." Bike for Your Life Project, 1998.

Brauer, Michael, and Christie Cole. "Cycling, air pollution exposure and health: An overview of research findings." Presentation given at VeloCity 2012, Vancouver.

Clean Air Partnership. "Bike Lanes, On-Street Parking and Business: A Study of Bloor Street in Toronto's

Annex Neighbourhood." 2009. http://www.clean airpartnership.org/pdf/bike-lanes-parking.pdf.

Harvard Health Publications. "Understanding the Stress Response." *Harvard Mental Health Letter* 27, no. 9 (March 2011): 45.

Hood, Sarah B. *Practical Pedalling: A Companion for Everyday Cycling in Toronto*. Toronto: Detour Publications, 1998.

Hurst, Robert. *The Cyclist's Manifesto: The Case for Riding on Two Wheels Instead of Four*. Guildford, CT: Falcon Guides, 2009.

Komanoff, Charles. "The bicycle uprising: remembering the midtown bike ban 25 years later." *Streetsblog NYC*. August 7, 2012. http://www.streetsblog .org/2012/08/07/the-bicycle-uprising-remembering-the-midtown-bike-ban-25-years-later.

Maus, Jonathan. "Study Shows Biking Customers Spend More." BikePortland.org. July 6, 2012. http:// bikeportland.org/2012/07/06/study-shows-biking-customers-spend-more-74357.

OECD/ITF. *Cycling, Health and Safety*, OECD Publishing and ITF, 2013.

Ottawa Humane Society. "Biking with dogs — be safe!" http://ottawahumane.ca/your-pets/biking_ with_dogs.cfm.

Partin, S.N., K.A. Connell, S. Schrader, J. LaCombe, B. Lowe, A. Sweeney, S. Reutman, A. Wang, C.

Toennis, A. Melman, M. Mikhail, and M.K. Guess. "The bar sinister: does handlebar level damage the pelvic floor in female cyclists?" *The Journal of Sexual Medicine* 9, no. 5 (May 2012): 1367–73.

Portland Bureau of Transportation. "Fact Sheet." http://www.portlandoregon.gov/transportation/article/407660.

Pucher, John and Ralph Buehler. *City Cycling*. Cambridge, MA: Massachusetts Institute of Technology, 2012.

Schwartz, James D. "Americans work 3.85 minutes each day to pay for their bicycles." *The Urban Country*. May 23, 2011. http://www.theurbancountry.com/2011/05/americans-work-384-minutes-each-day-to.html.

Reynolds, C.O., M.A. Harris, K. Teschke, P.A. Cripton, M. Winters. "The impact of transportation infrastructure on bicycling injuries and crashes: A review of the literature." *Environmental Health* 8, no. 47 (2009): 1–19.

U.S. Bureau of Transportation Statistics. "Pocket Guide to Transportation 2009."

Weddell, A., M. Winters, and K. Teschke. "Report of the Cycling in Cities Research Program." Vancouver, September 2012.

Contributors

I'm very grateful to all those quoted for sharing their invaluable insights. I'm thrilled and honoured to include their voices.

Lloyd Alter, managing editor, TreeHugger.com, @treehugger

Steve Brearton, Toronto writer and cycling advocate

Noah Budnick, deputy director, Transportation Alternatives, NYC executive director, San Francisco Bicycle Coalition, @transalt, @noahbudnick

Chris Carlsson, chriscarlsson.com and nowtopians .com

Andy Clarke, president, League of American Bicyclists, bikeleague.org/ridesmart, @BikeLeague

Mikael Colville-Andersen, urban mobility expert, CEO of Copenhagenize Design Co., copenhagenize .eu, @copenhagenize

Deadly Nightshades Bike Crew, nightshadesbike crew.blogspot.ca, @DNSbikegang

Clarence Eckerson Jr., director, Streetfilms, street films.org, @streetfilms

April Economides, president of Green Octopus Consulting, greenoctopus.net

Ken Greenberg, author of *Walking Home: The Life and Lessons of a City Builder*, Greenberg

Consultants Inc., greenbergconsultants.com,
@KGreenbergTO

Eric Kamphof, Curbside Cycle, curbside.on.ca,
@CurbsideCycle

Mia Kohout, CEO and editor-in-chief, *Momentum
Mag*, momentummag.com, @MomentumMag

Jared Kolb, executive director, Cycle Toronto, cycleto
.ca, @CycleToronto

Tania Lo, mother of two, COO and co-founder of
Momentum Mag, momentummag.com, @tania_lo

Lisa Logan, mother, photographer, and year-round
urban cyclist, @LisaLoganPhotog

Evalyn Parry, theatre-maker, songwriter, cycling and
history enthusiast, evalynparry.com, @evalynparry

Reba Plummer, worker-owner at Urbane Cyclist
Coop, @urbanecyclist

Jean-François Pronovost, vice-president development and public affairs, Vélo Québec, velo.qc.ca,
@VeloQuebec

Kelli Refer, yoga instructor and author of *Pedal,
Stretch, Breathe: The Yoga of Bicycling*,
@yogaforbikers

Étienne Roy-Corbeil, owner of Montreal's Dumoulin
Bicyclettes, dumoulinbicyclettes.com

Ryan J. Rusnak, AICP, city planner and 2012 Next City
Vanguard Class in Davenport, Iowa

Miriam Schacter, founder, danceFIT danceABILITIES

Canada, dancefitcanada.blogspot.com

Nancy Smith Lea, director, Toronto Centre for Active Transportation (TCAT), torontocat.ca, @TCATonline

Zack Stender, co-owner, Huckleberry Bicycles, huckleberrybicycles.com, @huckbikes

Lana Stewart, modalmom.com, @modalmom

Cory Sutela, current president of Medicine Wheel Trail Advocates, medwheel.org, and test development engineer for SRAM, sram.com

Kay Teschke, professor, School of Population and Public Health, University of British Columbia, cyclingincities.spph.ubc.ca, @kteschke

Todd Tyrtle, regulatory compliance consultant, riding for seven years in Vermont and Toronto

ACKNOWLEDGEMENTS

I'm deeply grateful to the many people who've contributed directly and indirectly to the creation of this book. This book would not have possible without a core team comprised of my editor, Jen Knoch, who provided the necessary support, encouragement, and deadlines to get me through the writing process; illustrator Marc Ngui, whose skill and dedication made him an absolute pleasure to collaborate with; art director Rachel Ironstone, who crafted the layout and design; and my research assistant, Jarret Ruminski, with whom I crossed paths at just the right time and who went above and beyond expectations. The additional and ongoing support of members of the ECW Press team has been fantastic.

A skilled and insightful group of friends and colleagues, a mix of new and veteran bike riders, were kind enough to participate as reviewers and provided invaluable feedback on an early draft. Thanks very much to Steve Brearton, Stephanie Power, Melanie Redman, Sarah Hood, Andy Clarke, and April Economides for their advice, assistance, and kind words. Thanks also to all those quoted throughout these pages, and those who have endorsed this collection of ideas and information that I've presented.

Throughout the research, planning, and writing of

this book, I bounced ideas off many lovely people, all of whom were kind enough to share their time, thoughts, and encouragement. In no particular order, I'd like to acknowledge the contributions of Daniel Egan, Eleanor McMahon, Nancy Smith Lea, Tammy Thorne, Alana Wilcox, Jason McBride, Eric Kamphof, Adria Vasil, Amanda Lewis, Trudy Ledsham, Gillian Goerz, Sam Higgs, Lina Cino, Pete Lily, Shamez Amlani, Michael Louis Johnson, Grant Mclean, Alex Jensen, Hayley Easto, Amish Morrell, Lake Segaris, Carl Hastitch, Chris Hardwicke, Howie Chong, Christina Bouchard, Reba Plummer, Patrick Brown, John Degen, Ian Flett, Elizabeth Radshaw, Anthea Foyer, Cassie Barker, McLean Greaves, Gilbert Li, Jason Diceman, Gabe Sawhney, Andrew Chiu, Josh Fullan, Jay Wall, Lisa Logan, Jessica Rose, Kristen Steele, Aunty Eva Simon, Roger Petersen, Martin Reis, Rick Conroy, Louis-Félix Binette, and Andrew Morton. Please insert your name here _____ if I've foolishly neglected to include you.

Additionally, I'm grateful to several organizations for their role in my completion of this book: the Ontario Arts Council for the Writers' Reserve grant; the Centre for Social Innovation, a co-working space where my office is located, which was usually deserted and quiet enough to get writing done over many a late night, weekend, and holiday; and Artscape at Gibraltar Point on Toronto Island for the weeklong residency that allowed me the headspace and solitude to complete the manuscript on deadline.

Finally, I'd like to thank all the amazing cycling pioneers, activists, and advocates who have worked tirelessly, from inside and outside institutions, and in countless creative ways, to carve the bike path we're now on — we've got momentum and it's thanks to your dedication. Ride on!

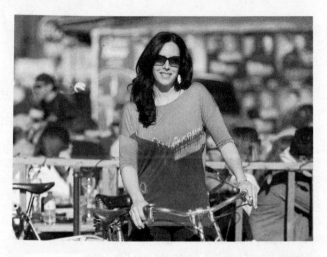

Yvonne Bambrick is an urban cycling consultant, event and portrait photographer, and executive director of the Forest Hill Village Business Improvement Area (BIA). She serves as a volunteer director on the Kensington Market Action Committee and as a member of the Metcalf Foundation's Cycle City Advisory Committee. She was the founding executive director of the Toronto Cyclists Union (now Cycle Toronto) and co-creator/coordinator of Pedestrian Sundays in Kensington Market. Yvonne is a regular contributor to *Momentum*, *Dandyhorse*, and *Precedent* magazines, and is the caretaker of Toronto's smallest park the Kensington Market Garden Car, a beloved neighbourhood icon and city-sanctioned public art project. And, yes, she does ride through Canadian winters!

Marc Ngui is a Toronto-based professional creator and one half of the art duo Happy Sleepy.

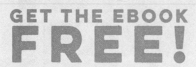

GET THE EBOOK
FREE!

At ECW Press, we want you to enjoy this book in